Tackle Football and Traumatic Brain Injuries

Tackle Football
and Traumatic Brain Injuries

Law, Ethics, and Public Health

Daniel S. Goldberg

Foreword by Christopher Nowinski

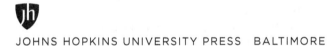

JOHNS HOPKINS UNIVERSITY PRESS   BALTIMORE

© 2024 Johns Hopkins University Press
All rights reserved. Published 2024
Printed in the United States of America on acid-free paper
9 8 7 6 5 4 3 2 1

Johns Hopkins University Press
2715 North Charles Street
Baltimore, Maryland 21218
www.press.jhu.edu

Library of Congress Cataloging-in-Publication Data

Names: Goldberg, Daniel S., 1977– author. | Nowinski, Christopher,
    foreword author.
Title: Tackle football and traumatic brain injuries : law, ethics, and
    public health / Daniel S. Goldberg ; foreword by Christopher Nowinski.
Description: Baltimore : Johns Hopkins University Press, [2024] | Includes
    bibliographical references and index.
Identifiers: LCCN 2024010340 | ISBN 9781421450117 (hardcover ; alk. paper)
    | ISBN 9781421450124 (ebook)
Subjects: MESH: Football—injuries | Brain Injuries, Traumatic | Chronic
    Traumatic Encephalopathy | Health Risk Behaviors | Health
    Policy—legislation & jurisprudence | Social Responsibility | Adolescent
    | United States
Classification: LCC RC451.4.B73 | NLM QT 260.5.F6 | DDC
    617.4/81044—dc23/eng/20240524
LC record available at https://lccn.loc.gov/2024010340

A catalog record for this book is available from the British Library.

*Special discounts are available for bulk purchases of this book. For more
information, please contact Special Sales at specialsales@jh.edu.*

Contents

Foreword

For all the advancements humanity has made in science, medicine, human rights, ethics, and protections for vulnerable populations, we still have blind spots. For example, did you know we probably let children get hit in the head more today than at any time in human history?

Most people agree that hitting children in the head is bad. But children are now exposed to billions of head impacts a year, in public, with their parents cheering, because the source of these head impacts is something believed to be good for children: team sports.

As a neuroscientist, I find this problematic. Inside a child's head is their brain, the most important possession they have in life. It will determine their intelligence, their success, and their happiness, as well as their ability to learn, cope, parent, and pursue their dreams. We know brain damage is bad, and brain disease is worse, and yet modern children can be hit in the head more than a thousand times a year in sports like tackle football.

Before organized sports, one would envision a child being hit in the head this frequently only in cases of abuse. Organized sports arose in the late 1800s—for college students—and became wildly popular. By the early 1900s, professional sports were born, as there was money to be made. There was nothing wrong with that—plenty of adults have dangerous jobs.

With this new opportunity for fortune and fame came incentives to become better at sports, which meant learning the games earlier in life. To get an edge, sports organizers began to recruit younger and younger children. But no one considered how the dangers of these sports might be different for children. Could children consent to the dangers? Could they understand the risk of lifelong injury? What do multiple head impacts do to a developing brain?

We now know what those head impacts can do. They can cause traumatic brain injuries, which can forever change how someone thinks, feels, and acts. More insidiously, they can cause chronic traumatic encephalopathy (CTE) a degenerative brain disease that progresses after the sports career ends. The most advanced stage of CTE usually causes dementia.

CTE was once called *punch drunk syndrome* because it was first seen in large numbers in boxers. Scientists studying CTE in the 1920s and 1930s predicted it would appear in other contact sports. But for some reason, both that discussion and the research stopped. When I signed up to play football in 1992 as a 13-year-old, no one was talking about CTE, and it had never been diagnosed in a football player.

In 2003, a traumatic brain injury ended my career with the WWE (World Wrestling Entertainment). By this time, I had been exposed to at least 10,000 head impacts playing football in high school and another four years at Harvard, where I played defensive tackle. When I developed headaches that would not go away, I started researching concussions and first learned about CTE. I could not believe I had been bashing my head so recklessly for so long without understanding where it could lead.

I felt people deserved to know the risks of contact sports, so I wrote *Head Games: Football's Concussion Crisis* in 2006. The NFL's response was that football does not cause CTE. I disagreed, and I cofounded the Concussion Legacy Foundation in 2007 to advance CTE research. CTE can only be definitively diagnosed by studying the brain after death, so in 2008 we partnered with the Boston University School of Medicine to create the UNITE Brain Bank, the first-ever academic center dedicated to CTE research. At that time, four NFL players had been diagnosed with CTE.

Fast forward to 2024, and the UNITE Brain Bank has diagnosed CTE in more than 700 of the first 1,000 football players studied. As a former football player, I am horrified by what is happening to these men. NFL stars who have been diagnosed with CTE include Junior Seau, Dave Duerson, Frank Gifford, Demaryius Thomas, Ken Stabler, Vincent Jackson, and John Mackey. One of those 700 was my former roommate and team captain my senior year at Harvard, Chris Eitzmann, who died fighting an extraordinary case of alcoholism.

In November 2023, the family of Wyatt Bramwell, who died by suicide at age 18 and had played football for 10 years, announced he was the first teenager diagnosed with stage 2 CTE. For context, this is the same stage Junior Seau was diagnosed with after 20 years in the NFL. Experts predict that with athletes getting bigger, stronger, and faster at every age, the physical impacts on the brain are only getting greater, and *CTE could become ever more common and more severe.*

Yet football is as popular as ever, and more than two million children under age 18—the age of consent—continue to play. Why? One reason is that aspects of the game have real value. Football teaches lessons about teamwork, overcoming adversity, and testing your limits in a way that other sports do not. Another reason is that the American tackle football industry fought back with a sophistication not seen since Big Tobacco.

You have undoubtedly heard these arguments, from football organizations or their doctors: football does not cause CTE; CTE is not a disease; CTE does not cause symptoms; the problems of former players are caused by alcohol, drugs, and missing the spotlight; players knew what they were getting into; children don't hit hard enough to get CTE; better helmets make football safe; concussion protocols make football safe; football is safer than it's ever been.

None of these statements are true, but you have heard these bad faith arguments promoted by an industry fighting for jobs, for profit, and for mindshare. Over the past 15 years, they have successfully weathered the storm. Today, a sport in which success and longevity are linked to CTE remains the most popular sport in America.

I'm not exactly sure what we should do—although I do advocate for many reforms through the Concussion Legacy Foundation—and I'm not certain who should be the ultimate arbitrator of what happens to football.

But I do know this: it is finally time for deep reflection on this CTE-creating machine. Daniel Goldberg has the experience and approach to guide us through this morass. We need to understand the role of football in our society through the lenses of bioethics, public health, history, and the law. We cannot stand by and let things continue as they are today.

I can promise you that no 5-year-old understands CTE and how it might impact his ability to pursue his dreams. He can't anticipate developing dementia in his 50s, bankrupting his family for his medical care, and leaving his children fatherless when they need him most.

I don't know what the answer is, but I know we need this discussion. This important book is a good start.

Christopher Nowinski, PhD
Founding CEO, Concussion Legacy Foundation
ConcussionFoundation.org

Tackle Football and Traumatic Brain Injuries

Introduction

In 1977, my family and I emigrated to the US from South Africa. I was nine weeks old. My parents, born and raised in South Africa, had made the difficult decision to leave everything they knew and loved. They did not believe that their children had a safe future in South Africa. By the mid-1970s, virtually everyone knew that the days of apartheid were numbered, and virtually no one predicted a bloodless transition of power. So we left.

Like most immigrants, we tried hard to assimilate into American society and culture. Sports was one way of doing so; and although it became obvious rather quickly that my brothers and I were not going to be leading any teams to victory, we could and did support the professional and college teams of our area. Of course, South African sports and American sports were not the same. In South Africa, rugby, cricket, and soccer were the dominant sports. To assimilate effectively, my family had to find analogues in American sports—games that we could understand quickly and easily. By that standard, the most obvious connection was between rugby and American tackle football. My father found it easy to follow the game of football. Moreover, we settled in football-mad South Florida, and the glory years of the Miami Dolphins (the early 1970s) were not far in the past. Thus, the relationship kindled.

Although there was no analogue in South Africa to major college sports, my father, an employee of the University of Miami, obtained tickets to the college football games. In 1984, only six years after we arrived in the US, my father and my older brother were at the Orange Bowl in Miami when the underdog Miami Hurricanes became national champions by narrowly defeating the Nebraska Cornhuskers. At this game, which is almost universally regarded as one of the greatest college football games of all time, my family's true passion for American tackle football was born. I was too young to attend the game, but I still remember waking up the next morning to my mother's thrilling whisper: "31 to 30; we won!"

Professional basketball did not come to South Florida until 1988. Professional baseball arrived in 1992. But football—football was there for us from the beginning. It was part of my immigrant family culture. I fed my love for history by reading histories of the game; I memorized players and statistics and spent many happy hours watching recordings of National Football League (NFL) games. My brothers and I grew up watching Dan Marino of the Miami Dolphins erase record books; we attended game after game at the Orange Bowl, as the University of Miami set records and won multiple national championships. Perhaps most significantly, I, my older brother, and my parents all became naturalized citizens in that very football stadium. In 1984, then vice president George H. W. Bush drove out to midfield and administered the oath of citizenship to approximately 10,000 people.[1] My family, save for my younger brother who had been born in the US, numbered among them.

Citizenship and football are literally intertwined for me.

I remained a passionate and dedicated football fan for decades. Tackle football is not just a deep part of US culture; it formed a critical part of the culture of my little family, who were virtually alone in the US with almost no extended family nearby. It was just us. And football. As my brothers and I grew into adulthood, football continued to bind us together. We could always talk about football, no matter how much we grew and changed. And so it continued.

In 2014, I was 37 years old and still loved tackle football. But that passion had been deeply impacted by my knowledge and expertise about the link between concussions and the sport. On a crisp fall afternoon, I was watching a game upstairs at home. My partner came into the room for a moment to get a book, and as she was leaving, she turned her head and asked, "How can you watch this stuff?"

She was not judging me. She was asking a plain and honest question: "Knowing what you know, how can you still watch this?"

Fifteen minutes later, I turned off the television.

I have not watched a game since.

×××

I wrote my first paper on ethics, concussions, and tackle football in 2007. In researching that paper, I was absolutely horrified to learn the story of a man named Mike Webster. During the 1970s, Webster had won four championships with the Pittsburgh Steelers and was widely regarded as one of the greatest offensive linemen of all time. I had watched him play for most of the 1980s and understood well the significance of his accomplishments in the sport. In writing my paper, I read feature stories about his life after he retired in 1991.

Eventually, I reached the point in his story in which the journalist Greg Garber recounted how Webster's headaches were so intense that he would beg his son to use a stun gun to shock him into unconsciousness.[2] It was the only respite he could get. Next, I read about Terry Long, whom I had also watched play for the Pittsburgh Steelers. Long died by suicide in 2005 after drinking antifreeze. Then my research led me to the story of Andre Waters, who had played defense for the Philadelphia Eagles, and whom, unlike Webster and Long, I had seen in the prime of his career. Just prior to writing my paper, in 2006, Waters died by suicide.

Even in 2007, these were not isolated stories. There were many others, none of which were especially hard to find. The more I read, the more disturbed I grew. The behavior of the NFL, the National Collegiate Athletic Association (NCAA), and their associates seemed extremely problematic. Conflicts of interest were rampant. Team physicians, trainers, coaches, and administrative officials repeatedly prioritized the best interests of the team over the health and well-being of individual players. Highly questionable scientific research and financial conflicts of interest were common; whistleblowers and objectors were silenced and punished; and outright denial of any long-term health risk caused by playing tackle football was the norm.

But as troubled as I was, I could not stop watching the game, although now I watched with significantly muted passion. I loved it too much. The game still knit together me, my brothers, and my father—it formed a crucible on which my immigrant family had forged its new identity as Americans. For the next six years, and while researching and publishing several more papers on the subject, I still found myself watching football on Saturdays and Sundays, poring over internet articles on my favorite teams, and tracking the game.

I did this until that day when my partner asked me a quiet, fateful question. Her question essentially rang a small bell inside my head; it made me realize that the passion and the spark was gone. I no longer loved football. I could no longer support it. Today I still cannot.

Between 2006, when I was researching my first academic paper on this subject, and 2024, the literature on the topic exploded. Concussions and collision sports are now almost daily news, and on a global scale. Countless newspaper and magazine articles have been published, as have dozens of books and hundreds if not thousands of academic and scientific papers. The US Congress has held multiple hearings on concussions and tackle football, and legislative and political bodies all over the world have become deeply engaged with the legal, ethical, political, and economic impact of the rising concerns over brain injury and collision sports. Advocates and organizations have forced FIFA, the international governing body for the world's most popular sport—soccer—to pay heed to the risks of play, although FIFA has repeatedly refused important measures that would likely reduce those risks.[3]

I dived deeply into the many works on the subject of concussions and collision sports. There was so much to learn, even more for someone who was trying to contribute to the national and international discussions on the subject. But the more I read, the more I became convinced that the general conversation on the subject, especially in the US context, were missing a key element: history.

I have professional expertise in law, bioethics, public health, and history. Even as a child, my deep research into the history of tackle football was no accident; I have always loved history. To the present day, I prefer to think historically—as a historian—about virtually everything. The subject of concussions and collision sports is no exception. I had already begun to draw on my historical training in my writings on the issue. But the more research I did and the more work I read from other scholars, journalists, and writers, the more I grew convinced there was a crucial historical angle missing from the national conversation. This angle begins with the understanding that American tackle football is an *industry*. Industries sell products, and sometimes these products can be dangerous. There is a very long history of industries using sophisticated ways to manage—and in many cases, obscure or deny—the health risks that their dangerous products pose. The key is that this history is not merely curious or interesting, like a knick-knack in a kitchen cabinet. Rather, the argument of this book is that this history is *essential*. We cannot make sense of contemporary debates regarding concussions and collision sports absent a solid grasp of this history. We also cannot plot a navigable course through these debates—and decide what the law and ethics require of us—without a sufficient understanding of the history of these industries and their impact on public health in the US.

×××

Since 2018, at least ten US states have introduced bills proposing an outright ban on youths under the age of 14 playing tackle football. While none of these bills has become law, momentum is plainly gathering in support of such a ban. This momentum is remarkable in a society in which tackle football is, by a fair margin, the most popular sport, as well as one of the most lucrative sports on the planet.

As one might expect, passions on the issue run high. In response to Massachusetts's 2019 version of such a bill, an opponent stated, "Banning youth tackle football is a tremendous overreach into the rights of parents to allow their children to play a game."[4] In January 2024, Governor Gavin Newsom, of California, threatened to veto a bill that would institute age cutoffs for tackle football, stating that he would "ensur[e] parents have the freedom to decide which sports are most appropriate for their children."[5] Framing the debate in terms of parental autonomy is important and is part of a larger history of resistance to public health regulations and reforms in the US. The most obvious example of this is the anti-vaccination movement in the US, which marshals similar rhetoric in defense of parental decisions to deny vaccinations for their minor children.[6]

The ethical question at the heart of this debate is difficult: To what risks should society permit parents to expose their children? Moral philosophers sometimes discuss the importance of easy versus hard cases, and there are many easy cases in which the answer to the above question is obvious. Permitting young children to attend school exposes them to elevated risk of contracting communicable diseases, but, at least outside of a global pandemic, few would suggest that the risks are severe enough to deny parents the right to enroll their children in school settings outside the home. On the other end of the spectrum, a parental right to permit their 7-year-old to operate an automobile seems obviously unacceptable from a risk perspective.

The hard cases make the ethical question difficult to answer. For example, motor vehicles cause tens of thousands of deaths and severe injuries every year. Developmentally, 16-year-olds often assess risks significantly less accurately than adults, which means that permitting them to operate an automobile likely elevates the risk of harms for themselves and others. On the other hand, there are myriad acceptable reasons why parents might permit 16-year-olds to operate an automobile. Is a decision to do so intolerable to the point that a society ought to eliminate the right to make that choice? Judging by the rates of injury, skiing is dangerous for children. Should parents be permitted to expose their children to such risks? Backyard trampolines send thousands of children to the hospital in the US annually, with approximately 0.5% of trampoline injuries causing permanent neurological damage.[7] Should they be banned?

There is a long history in the US of applying public health laws to regulate the risks of injury and death for youths and children surrounding the use of hazardous products. Judgments of whether these risks justify eliminating parental rights to choose which risks to expose their children to have their own history. But they continue to be at the core of the intensifying debate over the risks and benefits of participation in youth and adolescent football.

Although doctors and scientists have noted the concerning health impact of tackle football since the early twentieth century,[8] debates over whether children and youths should be allowed to play tackle football began to intensify at the turn of the twenty-first century. Starting in the late 1990s and early 2000s, major media outlets, including sports media outlets, produced harrowing stories depicting the suffering and deaths by suicide of retired players such as Webster, Long, and Waters. One of the greatest players of the 2000s, Junior Seau, died by suicide in 2012 via a firearm, but he had earlier driven his car off a cliff in 2010. (Seau's friends and family remain convinced this was in fact an attempted suicide, though Seau himself said he fell asleep while driving.)

As depicted in the 2015 Hollywood movie *Concussion*, the health issue exploded into full popular consciousness because of a paper published in 2005 in the journal *Neurosurgery* by a forensic neuropathologist at the University of Pittsburgh named Bennet Omalu.[9] In conducting an autopsy of Webster's brain, Omalu found extensive evidence of a disease named chronic traumatic encephalopathy (CTE). CTE is a devastating and progressive neurodegenerative brain disease that had typically been noted only in people subject to repeated brain trauma such as boxers or soldiers.

To find unmistakable pathological evidence of CTE in a retired football player was alarming, and the finding was front-page news in the most significant US newspapers. The shocking news about Webster's neuropathology, combined with the details of the suffering he endured, thrust the potentially devastating consequences of American tackle football into public consciousness. Over the next several years, a variety of news stories covered both the deaths by suicide of former professional players and some of the harrowing narratives players reported in being returned to play or practice by coaches, trainers, and physicians even after suffering serious traumatic brain injuries (TBIs) with significant acute effects.

One of the obvious and critical questions concerned the prevalence of serious brain injury. No one acquainted with the brutality of American tackle football doubted its capacity for harm. But if play posed serious risks of long-term and severe neuropathology to adults, the stakes of play were much higher for the 4–6 million youths and adolescents who play the sport. This book is concerned both with framing these debates in proper historical context, as well as issuing recommendations for how public health laws can be used to allocate the risks and benefits in ways consistent with our ethical obligations to each other and to vulnerable groups such as children.

The central argument of this book is as follows:

American tackle football is an industry. Like many industries, the products the tackle football industry sells are dangerous to those who participate (in this case—those who play it). If the true scope of the danger and the costs to society of caring for injured participants were to become widespread and public knowledge, the profitability and perhaps even the viability of the industry would be at risk. Therefore, like many industries, the tackle football industry has consistently worked to mask the health hazards involved in playing football. Moreover, they have used a particular tool that has proved highly effective for many industries in achieving this subterfuge: the Manufacture of Doubt. Fortunately, we can use public health laws as a tool for countering the Manufacture of Doubt, and we have ethical obligations to do so.

In chapter 1, I will sketch a broad outline of the history of this Manufacture of Doubt, and I will explain why it matters and how it frames the analysis of the book. Essentially, what is needed is a primer for how to think about the legal and ethical problems posed by injury (especially brain injury) and collision sports. This primer is just one among many— there are lots of useful and productive ways to think about these complex problems. Nevertheless, the argument of this book is that a basic familiarity with the history of regulated industries and their intersection with public health is needed both to understand the contemporary debates and to move forward with fair and equitable policy solutions.

Chapter 2 delves deeply into the Manufacture of Doubt, explaining its modern roots in regulatory, public health, and occupational histories. The chapter then specifies a number of key identifying characteristics of the scheme and grounds them conceptually. Chapter 3 applies that analysis to the American tackle football industry, demonstrating how the industry has manufactured doubt regarding the links between play and significant population health harms.

Chapters 4 and 5, respectively, take up two particularly important identifying characteristics of the Manufacture of Doubt: conflicts of interest and unreasonable demands for proof of causation. As to conflicts of interest, chapter 4 draws on the current, significant body of work articulating the most useful conceptual framework for thinking about such conflicts and then advances arguments applied to the tackle football industry. The chapter explains why, under ordinary epidemiologic standards, conflicts of interest are population health hazards and must be countered via law and policy solutions. Chapter 5 considers arguably the most important tool used by regulated industries to manufacture doubt, at least in the twentieth century: questioning causation and issuing unreasonable demands for proof of causation. Exploring further the evidence of this practice by the American tackle football industry introduced in chapter 3, chapter 5 critiques the script, and the tackle football industry's use of it, based on a fundamental principle of public health: the precautionary principle. This principle provides the epistemic warrant for public health action in general, including and perhaps especially public health law interventions aimed at advancing social and health justice.

Those public health law approaches are the central subject of chapter 6, which is also the longest and final chapter. Chapter 6 issues four policy recommendations intended to address the population health and ethical problems explained in the first five chapters. These recommendations aim to capture the power of law as a major social determinant of health. Chapter 6 details each of the recommendations with analysis and argument and also rebuts the most likely objections.

The book concludes, as this introduction begins, with some personal ruminations. As the saying goes, the personal is political. Part of my motivation in pursuing this topic is reflected in the statement attributed to the great Rabbi Tarfon, "It is not your duty to finish the work, but neither are you at liberty to neglect it."[10]

1

Public Health History and the
Manufacture of Doubt

In the debate over the ethical propriety of American tackle football, some observers are astonished that, for example, parents would willingly expose their children to a very real risk of long-term injury. Similarly, the fact that high school and college football in the US largely proceeded as scheduled during an out-of-control pandemic proved difficult to fathom for many, even as significant numbers of college players ended up testing positive for COVID-19. Obviously, parents and school officials who permitted such play might well weigh the state of the evidence differently, but such a statement of permission is really a series of questions masquerading as an answer.

1. *Why* do so many informed and perceptive stakeholders weigh evidence so differently?
2. *What* is at stake in the weighing?
3. *What* are the standards to be applied in making the measurement?
4. *Who* is to adjudicate the interpretation of those standards?

These are the fundamental questions with which this book is concerned. One theory that can frame possible answers is known as "deep play." Deep play is a concept first described by British philosopher Jeremy Bentham and further developed by anthropologist Clifford Geertz to explain why some games are of special significance to a given society.[1]

While virtually all human societies play games of some kind, the meanings of the games that are especially important can reveal important insights about a society.

Geertz labels these special games "deep play." Furthermore, many of these games seem to center ritualized forms of violence. Thus, in the US, American tackle football[2] is an example of deep play. In Canada, Finland, Sweden, Germany, the Czech Republic, and Russia, ice hockey is deep play. In most countries of the world, football ("soccer" in the US, and hereafter referred to as "international football" to distinguish it from the version played primarily in North America) is the central example of deep play. All of these sports involve collisions between participants moving at significant speed. As literature professor Natalia Cecire notes, "Deep play is enacted on bodies, human or animal, that will be violently sacrificed for this art."[3]

The very fact that American tackle football is deep play may go some way to explaining how people can weigh evidence so differently and reach such different conclusions on the ethical permissibility of exposing vulnerable groups to the risks of injury posed by collision sports. Similar observations can and have been made with regard to deep play in other societies in which collisions, combat, or related forms of violence are prominent. Although comparative analyses are always useful, the local, particular relationship between deep play and the communities to which it is attached makes exhaustive cross-cultural work quite difficult. Therefore, this book focuses on American tackle football.

The violence of deep play in general and collision sports in particular is important for another reason: it recommends a particular framework for ethical and social analysis, one rooted in a concept known as "structural violence."

Structural Violence

Drawing from liberation theology and peace studies movements, the concept of "structural violence" has been increasingly utilized in health policy and politics:

The term "structural violence" is one way of describing social arrangements that put individuals and populations in harm's way. The arrangements are structural because they are embedded in the political and economic organization of our social world; they are violent because they cause injury to people (typically, not those responsible for perpetuating such inequalities).[4]

Sometimes structural violence is literal, physical violence. But in many other cases, structural violence causes injury and harm through the constant force and pressure of social institutions. There are a variety of powerful social forces that converge in the modern world to create and sustain structural violence. One such factor is racism and in particular the linkage between histories of racism and economic gain. Although it is almost impossible to calculate precisely, economists and historians have estimated the value of chattel slavery in the many trillions of dollars. The economic engine of chattel slavery helped transform the US from "a colonial, primarily agricultural economy to being the second biggest industrial power in the world—and well on its way to becoming the largest industrial power in the world."[5] In a non-US context, Holocaust historian Götz Aly has argued persuasively that part of the reason why millions of Germans accepted the horrors of the Third Reich was because of the massive riches the Nazis acquired through subjugation, oppression, and attempted genocide.[6] This is in part why contemporary social theorists have devised the concept of racial capitalism, to explain how it is that organized and systematic racism has consistently been turned to enormous capital in the Western world.[7]

Racism and capitalism are therefore examples of social forces that are important causal factors in determining which communities enjoy preferential access to social factors that are themselves important determinants of health outcomes.[8] Another plausible example of a root cause that tracks historical patterns of domination and oppression is stigma. Stigma occurs when the in-group marks an out-group as deviant on the basis of a shared demographic characteristic. Because in-groups are by definition more empowered than out-groups (otherwise they would not be "in"!), stigma as a social process fundamentally reflects power relations in any given community.[9] The status loss and adverse social consequences of stigma can be devastating, and there is abundant evidence that stigma functions as a strong and independent determinant of health outcomes. As we will see, stigma and doubt of the extent of participants' injuries (sustained during play) has a long history both in occupational health and in collision sports in particular. Because stigma too is, at its root, a function of social power, stigma is best conceptualized as a structural force that exerts profound influence on many other important social determinants of health.

Racism, capitalism, and stigma are powerful components of structural violence. In turn, these forces are upstream determinants of all manner of social determinants of health, such as safe housing, educational attainment, employment opportunities, and safe working conditions, etc. These root causes of structural violence are critical to understanding both the unequal implications of harm caused by collision sports and the legal and policy priorities for interventions intended to ameliorate such harm. These priorities will be detailed in chapter 6, but for now, the key is to situate debates over collision sports and population health harm in the context of structural violence and the inequalities fueled by structural violence.

What does it mean to say that structural violence often operates through "institutions"? Which institutions? And how are these institutions connected to broad social structures? How do institutions "structure" social life in ways that cause harm to populations (some more than others)? This book is primarily concerned with a set of institutions and structures that center regulated industries. In the US, tackle football is not merely deep play. It is also an industry. Although this book is largely concerned with tackle football in the US, different sports may qualify as an industry in other places around the world. In Canada, ice hockey is an industry. In the United Kingdom, international football is an industry. And many of these industries are global in scale, as their status as Olympic sports demonstrates.

But what makes any particular business enterprise an industry?

American Tackle Football as a Regulated Industry

One classic formulation defines an industry as "any grouping of individual . . . businesses which is relevant when we study the behavior of any one such business."[10] Moreover, industries tend to be composed of businesses that share a "chief characteristic," such as similar manufacturing processes, technical resources, and backgrounds of experience and knowledge.[11] As applied to professional tackle football in the US, each of the 31 teams is without question its own independent business, as a matter of both law and fact. Yet, the teams share a number of these "chief characteristics" and interests that collectively make tackle football an industry. But the tackle football industry is not limited to the 31 professional teams; many other entities and organizations participate in the industry, including the NCAA, state high school athletic associations, Pop Warner (the largest oversight body for youth tackle football), USA Football, and so on.

However, what matters is not merely that tackle football in the US is an industry. What makes a historical approach so critical is that tackle football in the US is a *regulated* industry. A regulated industry is simply one in which "government has exercised the power to limit entry into or exit from the business, regulate the type or amount of a product or service offered, set the price and quality provided, and determine the sale terms and level of profits allowed."[12] Some industries go unregulated, either for a specific period of time, or indefinitely. Others may be strictly regulated at one point in time but may then be "deregulated," whereby government control over the industry is relaxed. The reason that the regulatory status of an industry matters is simply because government involvement has an enormous impact on the commerce and activities of the businesses in any given industry. In an unregulated or very lightly regulated industry, businesses have much more freedom to make decisions and behave in ways that serve their interests (often the maximization of profits). The reasons why governments in general and in the US in particular do or do not regulate a given industry can be quite complex. But one of the most obvious justifications for regulating an industry is to protect the public from harms associated with the commercial activities of the industry. When an industry tries to sell products or engages in activities that harm or threaten the public's health, a local, state, or federal government often intervenes and regulates the industry with the intention of eliminating or at least minimizing the health risk associated with the product.

This harm-based justification for regulation is a common one in US history. Industries have repeatedly entered products into the stream of commerce that are harmful to public health, and governments have tried to regulate them. Especially well-known examples include industries selling lead, vinyl, asbestos, automobiles, pharmaceuticals, and, of course, tobacco. Pharmaceutical products present a particularly interesting case study because they remained largely unregulated by the US Food and Drug Administration (FDA) until the early 1960s. Prior to 1962, the major law that governed the marketing and sale of pharmaceutical products, the Food, Drug, and Cosmetic Act, had last been amended in 1938. It said that pharmaceutical companies could legally sell their products "if the FDA didn't act within 60 days to prevent its marketing."[13] The FDA also lacked the ability to enforce good manufacturing processes. Although Senate hearings began in 1959, the thalidomide tragedy that unfolded over the next two years galvanized the legislators and changed regulatory history. Thalidomide is a sedative that began to be prescribed to pregnant women, largely in Europe and Canada, as a treatment for morning sickness. The drug was not authorized for sale in the US only because FDA medical officer Frances Kelsey, on the basis of insufficient evidence of safety, refused to approve the drug application.

As it turned out, the drug caused serious birth defects, and the images of thousands of children born with "shortened, missing, or flipper-like arms and legs" shocked viewers in the US. Although the FDA had not approved thalidomide, the manufacturer nevertheless distributed the product to physicians and registered nurses, some of whom used the drug on themselves or pregnant partners.[14] Eventually, the Senate passed the Kefauver–Harris Amendment, which ushered in the modern era of pharmaceutical regulation in the US.

The point is that pharmaceuticals transitioned from a period of relatively light regulation to one with more significant governance, in part because of widespread public concern that the products marketed and sold by the industry were harmful. In addition, note that the thalidomide issues impacted highly vulnerable groups—pregnant woman, fetuses, and subsequently the infants and children showing the consequences of in utero exposure to the drug. Thus, not all groups are equally affected by the harms associated with any given industry's product or products, and regulators and policymakers have long considered the relative vulnerability of different affected groups in deciding whether and how to regulate. This has obvious relevance for tackle football in the US, since the overwhelming majority of participants are youths and adolescents: estimates suggest that approximately 5–6 million children aged 6–17 participate in tackle football,[15] of which only about 25,000 go on to play at the intercollegiate level, with even fewer—1,500 or so—playing in the NFL (the principal professional league in the US). But it is not simply in general terms that children are more vulnerable from a public health perspective; there are scientific reasons why youths and adolescents are more vulnerable to brain injuries resulting from collision sports. For one, brains are still developing during childhood and adolescence and are more vulnerable to injury. Another reason is that during childhood and adolescence, neck muscles are underdeveloped relative to head size,[16] which also makes head injury more likely. Thus, the population that forms the overwhelming majority of participants in the tackle football industry is vulnerable in multiple senses.

How do industries tend to regard the prospect of more vigorous regulation of their commercial activities? Occasionally an industry may actually desire stronger government regulation, as in the newly emerging artificial intelligence industry.[17] Nevertheless, in the history of public health in the US, most industries have generally resisted stronger regulation of their business and commercial activities. While there are many reasons for such resistance, the most fundamental one is cost. Compliance with stricter regulation costs time and money, as do restrictions on how products may be marketed and sold, to whom, and under what conditions. At the extreme, some products deemed excessively dangerous may essentially be regulated right out of the market, which obviously prevents a given company from profiting from the sale of the product. The pharmaceutical company Merck, for example, removed rofecoxib from the market voluntarily in 2004 after the results of a clinical trial suggested that the drug caused increased risk of heart attacks and strokes. Although the FDA did not explicitly take regulatory action, the near-certainty that they would do so, absent Merck's voluntary recall, prompted the pharmaceutical company to act. (Merck would go on to settle lawsuits brought against it for the sale and marketing of the product for US$5 billion.)

In summary, industries in the US have historically often sold products that pose a risk of harm. These risks have, sooner or later, forced governments to take regulatory and legislative action to protect the public from those risks. For well over 100 years, regulated industries in the US have typically sought to avoid such regulation or lessen the stringency of the rules imposed to govern the manufacture, marketing, and sale of their products. And here is where the history becomes especially important: avoiding or lessening the impact of regulation generally requires a sophisticated legal and political strategy. Regulated industries have taken up that strategic effort in earnest. Over time, these efforts coalesced into a set of "scripts" that increasingly came to govern industry behavior.

Regulated Industries, Social Scripts, and the Manufacture of Doubt

The idea of a social "script" originates in the social sciences. Scripts are essentially commonly expected behaviors and/or actions that are appropriate in specific social contexts. For example, in the scripts that tend to govern dining out at a restaurant, the server will expect the guests to request the bill after dessert is finished. "Scripts . . . enable *understanding* of situations . . . and they provide a *guide to behavior* appropriate to those situations."[18] Scripts, of course, are not destiny. Humans deviate from social scripts, but such deviations are often remarkable and sometimes bring negative consequences (e.g., the server and restaurant may eventually grow frustrated with guests that occupy a table for several hours after dessert is completed). Thus, while people can and do stray from scripts, such scripts are nevertheless quite powerful in shaping human behavior, giving rise to an entire literature across social psychology, cognitive science, and sociology generally labeled "script theory."

Dominant social scripts do not only shape individual behaviors. "Organizations present many predictable settings with reasonably predictable actions, events, and behaviors."[19] Scripts are therefore extremely important within organizations—and industries—and may also be helpful in explaining key aspects of organizational and industrial behavior.[20] This book details one set of dominant social and cultural scripts that regulated industries accused of selling harmful products have consistently deployed over the last century in the US. For reasons that will become clear, I refer to this set of scripts as the "Manufacture of Doubt." A wide variety of regulated industries that share little in common other than all being regulated industries have repeatedly behaved in ways consistent with and even predicted by the Manufacture of Doubt. Like other scripts, the Manufacture of Doubt is not a ghost in the machine. Regulated industries used and continue to use this complex set of legal, political, and social strategies because they work. That is, these tactics emerged and survived precisely because they repeatedly proved effective in meeting the economic, legal, and political goals of these regulated industries.

The central claim in this book is that contemporary ethical, legal, and political debates over collision sports that pose risks of traumatic brain injury (TBI) must be understood in light of these scripts, centering on the Manufacture of Doubt. Rooting these contemporary dilemmas in this history provides a number of insights that are critical both to a deep understanding of the current set of problems, and ultimately to conducting robust ethical and legal analyses that can guide policy and practice. While there is much discussion regarding the ethics of collision sports, especially as to youth and adolescent participation, the vast majority of these debates are conducted in *present* terms and contexts. As important as these discussions are, there is relatively little conception of the significance of the *history* of regulated industries' efforts to manage the economic and political risks posed by harmful or dangerous products. This history explains so much of the response from professional sports leagues and the proponents of collision sports for both adults as well as for youths and adolescents.

Chapters 2 and 3 take up the Manufacture of Doubt in earnest. Collectively, they explain the origins of the script, the continuous and various uses to which it has been put over its long life, and its application to collision sports. Equipped with a historically fluent lens, the analysis in this book moves on to consider some of the most prominent ethical and legal dilemmas central to debates over youth and adolescent participation in collision sports. Chapters 4 and 5 focus on two issues highlighted by the Manufacture of Doubt and important to current debates over collision sports and injury: conflicts of interest (COIs) and the role of what is called "the precautionary principle." As to COIs, regulated industries have intentionally and repeatedly developed relationships with people and institutions that enjoy a high degree of public credibility (e.g., scientists, physicians, local health agencies, etc.). These partnerships have proved highly effective in achieving regulated industries' individual and collective legal and political goals. These same kinds of relationships and resulting COIs are certainly present in debates over rights regarding TBIs and are therefore critical to any thorough analysis.

As to the precautionary principle and chapter 5, much of the argument regarding the ethical and legal propriety of participation in collision sports turns on (1) what the available epidemiologic evidence means, and (2) what the available epidemiologic evidence justifies (in terms of interventions). The precautionary principle is the basic idea that actors are justified in taking public health action in the face of existing but uncertain public health hazards. The principle is increasingly recognized as one of the core justifications for public health action in general. This is partly because determining epidemiologic causation—that a given exposure causes a particular injury—is extraordinarily difficult. Thus, the stricter the standard for causation we require, the less likely we are to implement public health interventions. The precautionary principle is critical because it provides a basis for relaxing that standard, thereby justifying public health actions in general that, on balance and measured historically, have produced much more benefits than harms.

The historical framework is especially important in thinking about the precautionary principle. Regulated industries have consistently seized on the difficulties of proving a causal link between exposure to their product(s) and health harms to delay public health action and justify the regulatory and political status quo. Chapter 5 explores these issues in some detail, which sets up the ethical and policy analyses and recommendations explored in chapter 6. Chapter 6 draws on concepts and methods concentrated in the field of public health law. The chapter offers four central policy recommendations for ameliorating the inequitable burden of TBI arising particularly from collision sports in which large numbers of youths and adolescents participate. The analysis will also explain why robust models of social justice demand focus on prevention-based approaches that address social and structural determinants of TBI. These structural factors are arguably more important than diagnostic and treatment-based clinical approaches that occur proximal or sub-sequent to an actual TBI itself. While high-quality care will always be needed to care for people who have experienced and live with the consequences of a TBI, narrow focus on treatment protocols leaves unaddressed critical larger questions regarding (1) the risks to which society is willing to tolerate exposing vulnerable groups, and (2) what interventions designed to eliminate or reduce the risk to acceptable levels are justified.

Scope of Injury and Population

Before proceeding to the detailed explication of the Manufacture of Doubt, it is critical to delineate the scope of both the injuries under consideration here and the primary populations in which the relevant injuries occur. As to the scope of injury, note that the risks of participating in collision sports cannot be limited to brain injury. Brain injury has dominated discussion on the ethics of collision sports for a variety of reasons. First, the consequences of severe neuropathology are frequently catastrophic, not simply for the former player but also for that player's friends, family, and associates. Second, in the West, and in the US in particular, the brain is widely understood as the locus of identity and personhood.[21] Historians and sociologists of the brain have long documented the ways in which modern Westerners are particularly enthralled by the brain and its role in human experience. Joelle Abi-Rached and Nikolas Rose go so far as to sketch the contemporary rise of what they term the "neuromolecular gaze,"[22] or the idea that we try to understand important social phenomena in terms of neuromolecular explanations and interpretations.[23] In a very real sense, we tend to perceive the essence of our selves—what makes us "us"—as residing in our brains. Hence the idea of brain injury caused by collision sports challenges our very ideas of what it means to be who we are as people, as workers, as intimate partners, as parents, etc.

Although there are benefits to focusing on brains and brain injury in context of the risks of collision sports, there are also drawbacks. The primary deficiency of this focus is that it tends to divert resources away from an upstream approach rooted in good public health practices, which emphasizes both prevention and attention to the social and economic factors that drive public health problems in general. Brain-based understandings of the problem tend to promote brain-based solutions; if the problem is the brain sloshing around inside the skill upon application of appropriate force, then the answer is to minimize that sloshing, say, via fancy new helmet technology. The latter intervention, of course, does not center the larger social question: Should vulnerable groups, such as children and adolescents, be participating in collision sports at all? Nor do brain-based approaches center tried and true public health practices such as harm reduction (i.e., replacing tackle football with flag football for children under the age of 14).

While chapter 6 will discuss these issues in more detail, arguably the greatest limitation of a focus on brain injury is that the risks of collision sports go far beyond brain injury. Moreover, the questions of causation that lie at the heart of this book are far less contested for many of these nonneurological injuries. The most well-documented class of injuries associated with collision sports are musculoskeletal and inflammatory in nature: joint, bone, muscle, tendon, and ligament injuries are relatively common across a variety of collision sports and can easily develop into chronic conditions that affect a participant's life for years, and even decades, after play ceases. Chronic pain, for example, is associated with tackle football,[24] and there is comparatively little dispute among health professionals that the increased rates of such pain are a direct result of participation.

It is understandable that the neurological health risks associated with collision sports in general and tackle football in particular dominate our attention. Given the stakes of brain injury, it is even defensible. What is not defensible is ignoring the broader health risks that are also associated with collision sports. Chronic pain alone is an enormous public health problem. It can and does have a devastating impact on the lives of those who suffer from it, and it also subjects people who live with it to significant stigma. Moreover, substance use disorders (SUDs) are comorbid, or commonly occur alongside, various kinds of chronic pain.[25] This statement of fact could potentially be used to stigmatize people in pain and/or people who use drugs, so it is important to be clear: the reasons that explain this association are complex, and they relate both to the supply of drugs and the demand (i.e., the reasons why suffering people seek out drugs, alcohol, and other substances). Noting that there are connections between collision sports, chronic pain, and SUDs does not imply any moral judgment of any kind for anyone affected by these associations. Rather, if the public health goal is ultimately to help people, reduce suffering, and improve health, it is essential to address without judgment or stigma the fact that long-term exposure to collision sports can trigger lifelong pain problems, which in turn make substance misuse more likely.

People who live with chronic pain and people who live with SUD are obviously not identical groups, but the point of the epidemiology is that these groups can and do overlap. Both groups are highly vulnerable and are subject to multiple and interlocking stigmas (addiction stigma, SUD stigma, pain stigma, disability stigma, gender stigma, racial stigma, etc.). While the stories of people in these groups is not the subject of this book, the fact that long-term participation in collision sports may cause chronic pain, and may also increase the risk of SUD, is a significant finding that has serious implications for thinking about the health harms of participation in collision sports for vulnerable groups. Therefore, as difficult as it might be to discuss these issues without further stigmatizing already marginalized people, it is necessary if we are to consider the full scope of health harms posed by participation in collision sports.

While a focus on brain injury is permissible, in thinking about collision sports as a public health problem, we cannot omit from the analysis at least some regard for the full scope of injury, disability, and health harms that people who play collision sports experience. A public health approach to the health harms of collision sports requires a broader lens than a focus on brain injury alone.

An ethical response to the scope of injury posed by participation in collision sports also has to address the relevant populations for analysis. In public health, identifying the "right" public or population is critical. Sometimes this is quite easy; if the public health problem is identified as "elevated rates of type II diabetes among a Latine population living in the Little Village neighborhood of Chicago,"[26] then the target population is obvious. However, at other times, identifying the "right" population can be quite difficult. For example, we might be able to save many more lives in the future if we reduced the amount of money we spend on emergency care at the present time. However, implementing this plan might mean that more people needing emergency care in the present would likely die. Who are the relevant "publics" here? People currently alive? If so, which people? Infants? Children? Adults? Or perhaps the right population is people currently alive who are more likely to need emergency care. Future people are also a relevant public; in fact, a great deal of the ethical arguments supporting prioritization of the world's climate emergency depend on the interests of future populations, many of whom have not even been born yet. Moreover, sometimes the group who is the subject of the analysis is not the subject of the public health intervention. Policy change, for example, is typically not targeted at the group who stands to benefit. In the example above of a Latine neighborhood in Chicago, the correct audience for policy change might be city council members or other public officials involved in local and municipal government rather than the population bearing the burden of the public health problem itself.

The key point is that figuring out the right group or public for analysis and/or intervention is often difficult and ethically complicated. How do these concerns apply to TBI and collision sports? The national and global conversation regarding TBI and collision sports was without question spurred most dramatically by American tackle football and the NFL in particular. Given the prominence of the NFL in global conversation and in scientific work on TBI and collision sports, there is an understandable tendency to center NFL players in scholarly work on the subject. But here the above question is relevant: Are NFL players the "right" group from a public health perspective? Should we focus our attention and resources on the approximately 1,500 NFL players? Or do other groups have a stronger claim to our attention? And if so, why?

One strategy that public health professionals often use to gain clarity on the scope of the population that should be prioritized is to think in the largest terms possible. Conceived broadly, who is at risk? The answer is: people who play collision sports, especially American tackle football. And who plays American tackle football? Answer: 1,500 NFL players and approximately 5–6 million youths and adolescents. In other words, well over 99% of people who play American tackle football are not NFL players—and the overwhelming majority of that 99% will never be NFL players. Accordingly, by the denominator alone, we could argue that our attention and resources should be devoted to the 99%—the youths and adolescents that play American tackle football. In addition, as mentioned above, there is clinical and scientific consensus that these same groups face heightened risks for kinesiologic reasons. In terms of both neurological development and kinesiology, then, youths and adolescents face risks that adult players may not face or may not face to the same degree.

The process of selecting the right public for analysis and intervention is rarely a simple correspondence with absolute numbers. We will have concerns of fairness and equity if we focus our attention only on what majorities experience as health concerns—this would tend to increase inequalities between the haves and have-nots.

Nevertheless, where we are principally concerned with injury, sickness, and impairment in the population exposed to the particular risk at issue, the composition of that population is both scientifically and ethically relevant. That over 99% of the people exposed to the risk are not NFL players is a good reason for prominently highlighting this figure in any ethical and legal analysis. This does not mean ignoring the exposures faced by the 1,500 NFL players. Their health is intrinsically valuable, and given the length of time they are exposed to the relevant

risks, as well as the severity and intensity of the risks, NFL players remain a group of significant interest. Moreover, the NFL is hugely important socially, culturally, and politically. Its role in shaping and sustaining
the Manufacture of Doubt related to collision sports is unquestionably
global, both literally and allegorically.

Thus, while the concept of vulnerability is complex, youths and adolescents who play American tackle football qualify in at least two basic
respects: (1) they constitute the overwhelming majority of the population exposed to the relevant risks; and (2) they face heightened neurological and physiological risks of injury of all kinds. Childhood is also
considered unique within epidemiology because exposures in childhood
can affect health across the life span—that is, many years later—and
can even have intergenerational effects.[27] For example, starting in the
1940s, pregnant women in the US were prescribed a synthetic form of
estrogen known as diethylstilbestrol, or DES. In 1971, researchers linked
DES to a form of cervical cancer; women who were exposed to DES in
utero (so-called DES daughters) are nearly 40 times more likely to develop the cancer.[28] But the relationship goes well beyond exposures to
known toxicants and carcinogens and is observable at the broader social
level as well.

In the late 1990s, a famous CDC–Kaiser Permanente study recorded
the frequency and consequences of exposure to "adverse childhood experiences" (ACEs).[29] The study indicated that the accumulated burden
of multiple ACEs had a dramatic impact on health across the life span
(figure 1).

The ACEs study is only a small part of a mountain of epidemiologic
evidence showing how early childhood exposures are critical to shaping
health decades and even generations after the exposure itself. Indeed, so
powerful is this body of evidence, it has given rise to a subfield of epidemiology called life course epidemiology. Life course epidemiologists attempt to unravel the lifelong impact of relevant exposures and conditions from prenatal to geriatric phases, and across generations as well.
(It is worth noting that one of the life course health outcomes that is

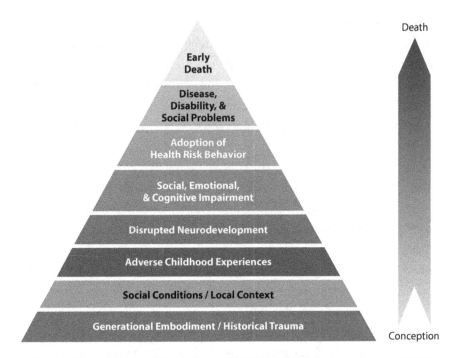

Figure 1. Mechanism by which Adverse Childhood Experiences Influence Health and Well-Being throughout the Life Span. (Source: The ACE Pyramid, Centers for Disease Control and Prevention, April 6, 2021, https://www.cdc.gov/violence prevention/aces/about.html.)

strongly correlated with exposure to ACEs is TBI, although that broader category of TBI does not necessarily imply participation in collision sports as the primary mechanism through which TBI results.)

Aside from the epidemiologic evidence, there are many philosophical traditions—including non-Western perspectives—that center children as worthy of special moral and ethical significance as well. Western traditions of medical and health care ethics consistently regard as different the dilemmas and problems related to the health of children. For example, the wishes and preferences of even mature adolescents regarding their health care are treated differently from the wishes of adults. With rare exceptions, a 13-year-old is not granted ultimate decision-making authority over their own health care. Informed consent must be provided by the authorized decision-makers (often but not always the parents). Part of the rationale for this differential treatment is the idea that children and adolescents lack the capacity to make truly informed and voluntary decisions. Similarly, as a matter of historical fact, children have received special attention in US public health laws and policies.[30]

The ultimate point of this analysis is to justify one central claim: any responsible public health analysis of collision sports and TBI must center children and adolescents. Primary justifications for this claim include: (1) children and adolescents make up the overwhelming majority of participants in American tackle football; and (2) children and adolescents are especially vulnerable to the lifelong health impact of exposure to collision sports.

Language Matters

Finally, before proceeding to the analysis in chapter 2, it is worth noting the different terms this book uses to discuss the various issues at play. The language we use matters a great deal, especially in thinking about policy. Sports medicine practitioners and injury epidemiologists have begun to move away from the term "concussions" for a variety of reasons. First, all concussions are TBIs. While many concussions can, at least in theory, be characterized as a "mild" TBI when compared to the severe neurotrauma that can result, for example, from a motor vehicle accident, there is increasing agreement among health care professionals and scientists that all TBIs can pose serious health risks, especially when they accumulate. The American Association of Neurological Surgeons notes that while "in most cases, a single concussion should not cause permanent damage," the very next sentence summarizes the danger of what is known as Second Impact Syndrome: "A second concussion soon after the first one does not have to be very strong for its effects to be permanently disabling or deadly."[31] There is an obvious tension between these two sentences—one concussion is generally fine, but two occurring in a short time frame can apparently cause severe disability or even death.

Second, while the term "concussion" has enduring relevance in popular discourse and understanding of head injuries, the term also comes with a significant amount of baggage flowing from the many decades when such injuries were thought to be relatively unproblematic. Given the current state of knowledge, this position is no longer defensible, if ever it was. Rhetoric and health communications studies make clear that the language we use has a dramatic impact on how we frame the risk of any given health concerns, including collision sports and TBI.[32] Moreover, how we frame the risks of brain injury in context of collision sports also goes a long way to determining the policy options and interventions we select or do not select.[33] Analysis of how we choose to frame the risks of public health hazards arising from regulated industries is at the core of this book. Thus, what language we use in discussing these risks matters a great deal.

Third, the increasingly preferred term in injury epidemiology, public health, and clinical practice is "traumatic brain injury." While language preferences among expert communities do not by themselves dictate terminology, it is advisable to root public health law and ethics work in the relevant scientific evidence bases. If communities of epidemiologists, public health scientists, and health care professionals that study and treat TBI in collision sports contexts prefer to use the term "TBI" over "concussion," that is a reason for doing so in legal and ethical analyses as well.

With the general framework and terminology at hand, the analysis can move to a detailed explanation of the Manufacture of Doubt and its application to American tackle football.

The Manufacture of Doubt and
Its Proponents

This chapter has two objectives. First, I will explain the Manufacture of Doubt. Second, I will highlight several especially significant and successful applications of the script. Chapter 3 will add a third objective: application of the script to the American tackle football industry's conduct regarding collision sports and TBI.

The Manufacture of Doubt is complex. I have already suggested that the best way to think of it is as a script or a set of scripts that regulated industries in the US have consistently used as a tool for achieving their regulatory, political, legal, and economic goals. While many of the specific historical details regarding the Manufacture of Doubt are beyond the scope of this inquiry, recall that the express argument of this book is that some kind of historicist or historically fluent framework is critical to making sense of our debates over collision sports and TBI. The historicist framework is also important for informing and shaping just and effective public health laws and policies. Part of the reason for the complexity of the Manufacture of Doubt are the ways the script seems to govern—and even predict—complex human behaviors at institutional and organizational levels. The reason industrial behavior is so often predictable on the basis of the Manufacture of Doubt is because the script is effective. Time and again, application of the script has assisted regulated industries in achieving many of their most important objectives.

Why? What makes the Manufacture of Doubt so effective?

Doubt in the Modern Era: Nineteenth-Century Changes

Doubt about causal links between a given injury or exposure and a health outcome are not new, especially when there are significant social consequences to the determination. Ancient communities hotly disputed causal attributions for epidemics where the suggested remedy was quarantine (which typically has a strong adverse impact on commerce). In seventeenth-century Rome, Italian physician and medicolegal expert Paolo Zacchia often testified about ways in which the body's physical signs undermined an injured person's causal claims.[1] Despite these important historical roots, the ways in which doubt is manufactured by sophisticated industries is a distinctly modern phenomenon. And the construction of doubt in the modern era has especially important roots in the nineteenth century.[2]

Although it is a cliché statement, the nineteenth century was a period of intense and rapid change, especially for the West. Industrialization, urbanization, and migration transformed the worlds of Westerners on both sides of the Atlantic Ocean. Labor and family patterns shifted in a variety of ways, and the social welfare state was born. As to medicine, Michel Foucault put it rather dramatically: the clinic is born in Paris in and around 1800.[3] Both the state of medical science and medical practice undergo enormous changes over the long nineteenth century, changes that in powerful ways structure ongoing and difficult experiences in the delivery, practice, and financing of health care and public health. Indeed, the very idea of social insurance provided by the welfare state is born during the nineteenth century, its implementation generally attributed to Otto von Bismarck, chancellor of Germany. Forensic medicine and science arise in the latter half of the century. Medical specialties begin to emerge during the last quarter of the century. Surgical theaters and hospitals alter their practices based on the emergence of anesthesia, sanitary practices, and shifting concepts of disease. Hospital architecture itself undergoes significant change.

And of course countless bloody conflicts engulf the world, many connected to colonialism and empire. Modern scientific racism, although not born in the nineteenth century, grows in popularity, regard, and impact. Eugenics dominates both lay and intellectual communities in the West, and by the end of the century its own popularity and reach was unquestionably transatlantic. In the US, state-sanctioned violence against a variety of minority groups, but especially targeting Black and Indigenous peoples, grows in scope and terror. Yet at the same time, emancipatory movements, especially among Black people and women, also gather force and power.

Ultimately, the full breadth and scope of the global changes during the nineteenth century are impossible to capture here. People living at the time were typically well aware of both the magnitude and pace of the changes, and they struggled to manage this anxiety. In the US and Great Britain, and arguably to some extent in most of Western and Central Europe, people searched for beacons, lighthouses in the fog and the chaos, upon which they could ground ideas and beliefs as true and enduring. Historians of science have long pointed out that ideas of truth change over time, and the middle decades of the nineteenth century mark one of these changes.[4] It is no coincidence that detective fiction as a genre and the field of modern forensic medicine is born in the mid-to-late nineteenth century The hope was that scientific processes could be used to investigate nature and reveal objective truth. In this, the nineteenth-century medical man is cast as the sort of somatic detective, able to ferret out the causes of a patient's malady and administer the appropriate intervention.[5] Sir Arthur Conan Doyle, the creator of the archetypal Sherlock Holmes, was trained as a physician.

In particular, people in the US were especially afraid of the deception of appearances.[6] Things might look okay on the surface, but the profound social dislocations of the time reduced people's confidence that their senses could be trusted. Scientific techniques paradoxically both weakened and strengthened these doubts; for example, people widely lauded the photograph as revelatory of truth. Yet, at the same time, people voiced significant anxiety over the ways that photographs could be altered or "doctored."[7] Coinciding with the immense popularity of Spiritualism in the late nineteenth century, entrepreneurs hosted seances and trumpeted the practice of spirit photography (by which ghosts and spirits could be shown on film); yet New York City prosecutors actually tried one of the most famous of these spirit photographers—William Mumler—for criminal fraud and larceny.[8]

Concerns that sick or injured people were feigning illness or "malingering" also began to increase over the nineteenth century.[9] A significant uptick in the written use of the word "malingering" during the late nineteenth to early twentieth century has been verified by indexing sources. More relevant for our purposes here is the extent to which doubt over the legitimacy of illness or injury complaints is consistent with the rise of regulated industries in the mid-to-late nineteenth century. Indeed, some of the earliest significant state and federal efforts to regulate corporations in the name of environmental and public health in the US can be traced to the last quarter of the nineteenth century. In part this is because many of these regulated industries were dangerous, both to their workers and to consumers. The railroad industry is a paradigm case of a Gilded Age hazardous industry. Even more important, for our purposes here, is the deep connection to doubt and its manufacture that one can find in the history of railway medicine and surgery.

Doubt and Regulated Industry: The Railroads

In tracing some of the origins of the Manufacture of Doubt, there is no question that the railroad industry is of special importance. First, by nineteenth-century standards, railroads were immense logistical undertakings, requiring significant capital, countless workers, and constant quality control (which was difficult by industrial processes of the time). Second, railways were capable of generating immense wealth. Third, they were quite dangerous to both workers and passengers (again judged by nineteenth-century standards—people alive at the time often regarded railways as dangerous).[10] Nate Holdren points out that "the early twentieth century US economy was rife with industrial violence,"[11] and injuries associated with railroads unquestionably constitute a significant component of this violence.

Judged by the size of the regulatory state today, state and federal regulation of the railroad industry in the late nineteenth century was light.[12] This gradually began to change in the first quarter of the twentieth century under the spate of Progressive approaches that sought to harness scientific laws and findings in the service of governance and civil society. But in the last quarter of the nineteenth century, railways were significantly less affected by a broad regulatory regime that governed their affairs.[13] As their commercial footprint grew in size and scope, railway corporations increasingly had to grapple with the relatively large number of their workers that had been injured in the course of their employment. At first, the railway corporations refused any responsibility for such injuries, but frustrated workers in the US turned to another weapon at their disposal. And this stick had a sharper end: litigation.

Historians of medicine and law have documented the connections between the high numbers of injuries experienced by mid-to-late nineteenth-century railway workers and a spurt in the growth of personal injury litigation arising in tort.[14] While railway litigation is not the sole explanation for the rise of malpractice and negligence-based lawsuits around the turn of the century, neither is it irrelevant.[15] Moreover, this situation, which was increasingly intolerable for the large railway corporations, is in a small way responsible for the particular structure of health care organization and delivery in the US to the present day.[16] Railway corporations actually mark an important point in the history when large American companies began to sponsor health care services for their workers. At present, approximately 54% of Americans obtain health insurance through plans provided by their employers.[17] While the history that led to this current state is complex and spans more than a century, it is fair to say that the railway corporations' decision to hire physicians and health professionals for the benefit of their injured workers is a watershed moment.[18]

Railway corporations hoped that by providing low-cost care directly to their injured workers, they could curb the workers' recourse to tort litigation. For many physicians in particular, this was attractive work, with the promise of an employer with deep coffers and a busy practice where much could be learned; the kinds of injuries produced by the immense mechanical and crushing forces involved in the operations of railways were of professional interest to many medical men of the time. Of course, the arrangement presented an obvious conflict of interest. Health professionals directly employed by railway corporations had financial incentives to please their employer. Contemporary decision scientists often term this particular problem "motivated bias," and it is extremely important both in the Manufacture of Doubt as a framework and specifically as to collision sports and TBI. Indeed, conflicts of interest are immensely important not just for collision sports and TBI, but for public health in general. Accordingly, it is the subject of chapter 4.

What is important here is to understand that many contemporary problems in public health and health care in the US have important nineteenth-century roots. Historians Alison Bashford and Carolyn Strange argue that "whether or not they make explicit links to the present, historically minded studies of public health confirm that past practices inhere in current perceptions and policies, which, like their antecedents, unfold amidst shifting amalgams of politics, culture, law and economics, in addition to increasingly sophisticated medical expertise."[19] This book explicitly adopts a historicist lens precisely because fluency with the public health, medical, and environmental histories helps explain so much of the contemporary debates regarding collision sports and TBI. The physician and novelist Michael Crichton wrote that "a person who doesn't know history is like a leaf that doesn't know it's part of a tree."[20] As distant as it may seem, ideas and events that began to bubble and change social life in the late nineteenth century are roots of the tree from which problems and questions surrounding collision sports and TBI sprout.

Indeed, railway health care presages other significant developments in health care policy to the present day. For example, Paul Starr, in his 1982 field-changing text, *The Social Transformation of American Medicine*, notes that American workers, well into the twentieth century, often mistrusted company-provided health care, and this was a major reason employers begin to shift to models of indirect provision of care after World War II.[21] Under these latter arrangements, companies contracted with insurers or third-party administrators to structure and deliver care, including reimbursement of providers. The extent to which this shielded American patients from the effects of conflicts of interest is debatable; the key point here is again that policy developments spurred in the nineteenth century continue to shape the structure of US health care to the present day.

But railroad workers were not the only population subject to injury from the railroad industry in the nineteenth century. Railroad accidents involving passengers were all too common in both the US and Great Britain. Trains are giant machines that move at tremendous speeds. The forces they could exert on human bodies were horrifying, and mass media of the period is absolutely filled with text and images of the carnage and trauma that railroad accidents could cause. Passengers sought recourse in tort litigation, and questions of injury, causation, and damage began to grow in importance alongside the growth in lawsuits. The railroad corporations therefore regarded their employee health care professionals as an obvious choice to serve their own needs in defending against personal injury litigation brought by injured passengers.

Railway physicians and surgeons thus spent much of their professional life in a forensic role. They needed to determine the etiology and nature of workers' injuries, both to provide quality care and to serve the commercial interests of their employers. They also served as expert witnesses for railroad corporations in tort litigation,[22] and therefore examined injured plaintiffs to discern the nature and scope of the patient's injuries, which in turn shaped decisions on whether to settle or go to trial, as well as questions regarding the possible damages and liability the corporation faced.[23] (As chapter 4 will discuss in detail, noting the ways in which conflicts of interest tend to shape human behavior does not require any character aspersions of individual people. We are all subject to the influence of motivated bias, and nothing about the professional practice of medicine insulates anyone from such influence.)

For both injured passengers and injured workers, railroad corporations had obvious incentives to manufacture doubt. As Holdren notes, company physicians "practiced medicine as surveillance of employees, for the financial benefit of businesses. Rather than providing care to the physical body of the individual injured person, these doctors provided care to the financial body of the corporation."[24] The railroads, in turn, countered that both passengers and workers had obvious incentives to puff up or even fabricate outright the existence and severity of the injuries they experienced. Railroads and railway physicians were most aggrieved by claims for damages arising from nervous disease and nervous injury, for they argued that many of these illnesses could not be correlated with material pathologies that could be detected by medical science of the time. Some physicians were especially convinced that passengers and workers were perpetuating a massive con, feigning illness and malingering commonly and with abandon. American neurologist Pearce Bailey wrote in 1898 that "the number of persons who demand compensation from corporations for trivial injuries, or whose claims are fraudulent . . . must be very large indeed."[25]

Railway physician Shobal Vail Clevenger wrote in 1889 that "the disposition to sham, to defraud, to play the hypocrite, to delude, to pretend, is an all too universal trait, but one that has been legitimately inherited from our most remote and beastliest ancestors. . . . Malingerers, as a rule, are of this low type, possessed of a species that links them to animals."[26] Fortunately, Clevenger wrote, skilled physicians should easily be able to detect malingering: "The physician familiar with a certain disease does not need rules for the detection of simulation, as feigned symptoms unfailingly strike him as grotesque."[27] British railway physician Herbert William Page in 1883 lamented "how easily, under the besetting temptations of railway injury, might a hastily expressed conclusion . . . have given an unscrupulous patient the opportunities of using his natural peculiarity for purposes of deception and fraud."[28]

Moreover, professional debates regarding the "reality" of passengers' and/or workers' injury complaints could be vicious. Danish-born British surgeon John Erichsen, who took a special interest in nervous disease and injury, found himself in a storm of controversy upon the 1866 publication of his treatise *On Railway and Other Injuries of the Nervous System*. In the book, he asserted that what was called "spinal concussion" or "railway spine" was in fact rooted in "organic" material lesions that were physically located in the nervous system.[29] Railway surgeons and like-minded colleagues rejected Erichsen's claim that a lesion somewhere in the spinal cord must somehow be responsible for cases of shock and nervous injury resulting from railway accidents. As Ralph Harrington notes, many late Victorian and Gilded Age physicians actually believed their patients' railway spine complaints even if they denied the existence of lesions in the nervous system that could explain it.[30] Opinions on the subject were nevertheless divided; there were no shortage of doctors in both the US and the UK who were much more skeptical of such claims (railway physicians prominent among them, of course). Then, as now, the odds of being accused of feigning illness or malingering were deeply affected by one's gender, race, and class.[31]

We can draw more connections between railway spine, the origins of the Manufacture of Doubt, and contemporary debates over collision sports and TBI. Historians have referred to the diagnosis of "railway spine" as nineteenth century whiplash.[32] Whiplash is notorious in the US in particular as a claimed neurological or spinal injury resulting from a motor vehicle accident. Just like railway spine, whiplash is widely associated with questionable personal injury litigation and unscrupulous plaintiff's attorneys. Harrington observes that

> the doctors concerned with railway spine . . . recognized from the outset that the clinical history of "railroad cases" could not be separated from the medico-legal issues in the courtroom. The drama of railway spine took place, not solely within the closed circle of the doctor-patient relationship, nor in the carefully controlled realm of the medical laboratory, but in the public arena of the court of law.[33]

Just as the railroad industry sowed doubt regarding the causal connections between their products and the kinds of severe trauma that can result from use, so too did it seek to undermine the validity of personal injury claims resulting from railway accidents. Moreover, whiplash arises in context of the automobile industry, which has been a major player in the twentieth century Manufacture of Doubt. And many of the strategies used by both parties—separated by almost a century—center on undermining the claims of causation between use of the product and the resulting harm. Much more will be said about causation below. Nevertheless, the parallels are unmistakable.

Finally, physicians filled hundreds, if not thousands, of pages in medical journals and treatises arguing over the anatomical correlate that could explain railway spine. Erichsen's work was controversial not because he ascribed a physical cause to railway spine, but because he rooted the "seat of disease" in lesions in the spinal cord itself. Most physicians doubted any such neuroanatomical pathology was associated with railway spine or spinal concussion. Why the existence of an anatomical dysmorphology was deemed so critical is important, but it is too complex a story to cover in detail here. The basic idea is that nineteenth-century ideas of scientific and medical truth began to hinge on the discernment of material pathologies inside the human body that could be clinically correlated with the patient's illness complaints.[34] The absence of such pathologies did not guarantee medical doubt, but there is sufficient evidence from which to conclude that doubt of such "lesionless" illnesses was much more likely than for illnesses with obviously connected "morbid" pathologies.

For our purposes here, the point is that debates over neuroanatomical changes and insults arising from injuries involved in using the regulated industry's product are a prominent feature of both nineteenth-century railroad disputes and twenty-first-century debates over collision sports and TBI. This similarity is fascinating and important. Neuroanatomical evidence was, and is, almost universally deemed critical in both discourses, even though they are separated by over a century. Indeed, the current round of arguments about American tackle football and TBI exploded as a direct result of new neuroanatomical evidence: forensic neuropathologist Bennet Omalu's autopsy of former NFL player Mike Webster's brain. And debates over the quality and implications of the collection of neuroanatomical evidence developed by Ann McKee and colleagues has occupied an enormous amount of the debates surrounding TBI and tackle football.

At least part of the reason for this seemingly repeated emphasis on neuroanatomy in cases of alleged industrial harm is the neuromolecular gaze.[35] This refers to the late twentieth-century tendency to regard as convincing neuroscientific and neurobiological explanations for human behavior and other social phenomena. Contemporary ideas of scientific and medical truth are strengthened when neurobiological explanations are provided. One influential study found that an identical piece of writing was more persuasive when it was accompanied by functional magnetic resonance imaging (fMRI) pictures.[36] For well over a century, in the US in particular, people have deemed neuroanatomical evidence an important marker for scientific and medical truth. Moreover, public health hazards arising from products sold by regulated industries have repeatedly been a key focus for disputes over such evidence.

The claim in this section is not that the social script known as the Manufacture of Doubt begins out of nothing in the context of the late nineteenth-century US railroad industry. In fact, the reason for discussing the social ruptures of the long nineteenth century is precisely to indicate the insidious growth of doubt in the modern era. Yet there is no question that these larger social contexts of doubt manifest in a particular way within the railroad industry's attempts to manage the liability risks and damages claimed by injured workers and consumers. Moreover, the size and sophistication of the railroad industry meant that it was enmeshed with other growing ventures that were also concerned with the truth of illness and injury complaints. The most obvious of these is the insurance industry, which experienced rapid growth in the first quarter of the twentieth century as multiple types of insurance policies began to be sold (i.e., property insurance, sickness insurance, workers compensation, etc.).[37] One of the most vehement and historically significant expositors of malingering in the modern era is a man named Sir John Collie. Collie, a Scottish physician, served as medical examiner both to the London City Council and the Metropolitan Water Board, and also for at least three insurance companies and a shipping interest. In 1913, he published an influential "pamphlet"—of 340 pages—titled, simply, "Malingering and Feigned Sickness."[38]

Doubt begins to be manufactured in important ways within the rise of railway medicine and railway litigation. The resulting debates and contests track across medicine and health care, into occupational and public health, as well as law, at legislative, regulatory, and judicial levels. The Manufacture of Doubt is a deep and powerful social script. Some of its power comes from its breadth and the many social sectors and communities it touches. Yet, within the script twentieth-century actors in particular began to develop focused strategies that can be specifically applied in the right contexts to nourish doubt. The best example of this is the increasing emphasis on causal insufficiency, which will be covered below.

Although there is evidence that the railroad industry would continue to manufacture doubt into the twenty-first century, other industries pick up the mantle and enter the regulatory fray. The remainder of this historical scan will provide some key details in the Manufacture of Doubt beyond those important foundations perceptible within the context of railroads. Other industries that have been analyzed by scholars include, but are not limited to: mining, chemical, lead, vinyl, automobile, pharmaceutical, tobacco, and oil and gas industries. A few examples suffice to make the point and apprehend the key details of the Manufacture of Doubt.

Silicosis, the Mining Industry, and the Manufacture of Doubt

Silicosis is a deadly lung disease that is caused by inhaling silica dust. As historians David Rosner and Gerald Markowitz note, the disease exploded into prominence directly because of the massive industrialization of the nineteenth and early twentieth century. "Silicosis was an industrial disease whose roots were in the changing production methods—automation, assembly lines, and modern notions of efficiency—that had produced the affluence that twentieth-century Americans had come to believe was their birthright."[39] The social reform movements of the late nineteenth century focused on the connection between substandard labor conditions and ill health. Within this context, early twentieth-century welfare reformers, physicians, public health officials, and statisticians began to take notice of what one insurance company statistician in 1908 called the "Mortality from Consumption in the Dusty Trades."[40] By the late 1910s, physicians and officials in the US began to understand silicosis as a distinct industrial disease rather than simply a form of tuberculosis. Rosner and Markowitz explain, "The studies of British workers in South African gold mines attracted widespread attention to the devastating effects of industrial dusts and specifically silicosis on the health of the work force."[41]

Ironically, public health officials resisted this conclusion, but the work of Frederick Hoffman, the author of the 1908 report on the "Dusty Trades," filed a report in the early 1920s for the Vermont Department of Labor. Hoffman showed that "despite nearly identical rates in 1896, the granite cutters' rate [of 'tuberculosis'] rose 400 percent, while the general population's declined more than 50 percent."[42] By the end of the decade, "public health investigators had documented the dangers posed by silica dust in a host of industries."[43] In 1931, a private organization, the National Safety Council, hired Charles-Edward Amory Winslow, a professor at Yale and arguably the most prominent public health leader in the country, "to prepare a report on sandblasting and the danger of silicosis."[44] At the same time, Rosner and Markowitz point out, lawsuits filed by injured workers were steadily rising, and the various industries implicated in silica dust exposure were marshaling resistance both to the litigation and to Winslow's report. The foundry industry in particular objected to the draft report, sending "hundreds of telegrams and letters . . . demanding the right to inspect and amend the report."[45] In an early manifestation of the Manufacture of Doubt, the foundry industry's negotiations with the National Safety Council succeeded in influencing the publication of the report: two papers were published in the scientific literature. The first, which included Winslow as author, appeared in a German journal *Archiv für Gewerbepathologie und Gewerbehygiene* (Archive of Industrial Pathology and Industrial Hygiene).[46] The article explicitly articulated a connection between sandblasting and silicosis. The second article appeared in the *American Journal of Industrial Hygiene*. It excluded Winslow as an author, said nothing about the connection between foundry work and silicosis, and mentioned the word "silicosis" only once.[47]

Like the railroad industry, which became more and more interested in manufacturing doubt as a response to the increase in personal injury litigation arising out of worker and consumer use of the product, the mining and foundry industries responded the same way when hit with significant litigation. "In New York State alone, the foundry industry faced over $30 million in lawsuits in 1933."[48] The insurance industry fulminated over these lawsuits and strongly pressured state and federal governments to address their liability via inclusion of industrial diseases into workers' compensation schemes.[49] In 1936, news broke of the disaster at the Gauley Bridge in West Virginia, in which as many as 1,500 workers died due to silica dust exposure while working on a tunnel project.[50] This event ushered silicosis into national consciousness, and the US House of Representatives responded by holding hearings. During Franklin Delano Roosevelt's second term, Secretary of Labor Frances Perkins took a special interest in the silicosis problem. Yet she realized that massive and well-organized industry opposition made new federal legislation that protected workers impossible. Department strategy thus turned to getting industry to accept voluntary standards, which required significant industry involvement. Rosner and Markowitz write, "Significantly, of the twenty-six new planning committee members invited to the [inaugural] meeting, fifteen represented various affected industries and only three represented labor."[51]

The sequence of events and the broader picture it represents in the Manufacture of Doubt is important. Chapter 1 notes that one of the primary objectives of the Manufacture of Doubt is to create a vacuum in which governance of the regulated industry's conduct and commercial activities is kept to a bare minimum. By the time Perkins became involved in 1936, the industries implicated in the silicosis debate had already accomplished one key objective in the vacuum: they had managed to eliminate the possibility of federal legislation, at a rare moment in US history in which federal legislation of social and industrial problems was relatively vigorous (the New Deal).

Indeed, it is typically difficult to enact major federal legislation, let alone legislation on a contested issue, with vehement, sophisticated, and well-funded opposition from a regulated industry. Moreover, regulatory bodies (agencies) exist, at least in part, for the purpose of providing specific, timely, and ongoing governance of industrial behavior. Thus, where legislation is unlikely at the federal level, the obvious next step, demonstrated neatly in the silicosis case, is to turn to agencies and regulation to curb population health hazards arising from occupational and industrial exposures. This is exactly what the Roosevelt administration tried in 1936. But industrial actors are sophisticated—even while moving to negate the slim possibility of legislative action, they are positioning themselves for the real battle: the regulatory fight. The story of silicosis thus offers up a key plank in the Manufacture of Doubt as applied in the regulatory sphere: the phenomenon of regulatory capture.

Regulatory Capture

Regulatory capture occurs when "agencies tasked with protecting the public interest come to identify with the regulated industry and protect its interests against that of the public."[52] To understand the phenomenon and why it is such a serious problem for public health in general, it is necessary to back up a bit and explain the role of agencies and regulations in US law and politics. Say that the US Congress has decided that it wants to pass a comprehensive workplace safety law. It is literally impossible to craft a law that provides specific guidance to the thousands of different kinds and sizes of employers in the US. Each of these employers will need to know how to interpret the requirements of the law and how the requirements apply to the specific commerce and business in which they are involved. Moreover, it is extremely unlikely that many of the legislators who voted for the new law are workplace safety experts. Indeed, none of them may possess such expertise. That expertise is critical to providing the specific guidance needed to implement the legislation.

To oversimplify, we can say that legislators enact the law, while regulators implement it. Indeed, in virtually every significant piece of legislation, there is a part known as an "implementing provision," in which the legislature formally directs a given regulatory body to create the rules and regulations needed to implement the legislation. Thus, some scholars have argued that regulatory law (or, as it is also termed, "administrative law" because such laws tend to govern how legislation and statutes are administered) is the principal form of contact most Americans have with "law" on a daily basis. Everything—from the safety features on the automobiles and public transit we use to the size of the offices, number of bathrooms, and fire exits in the buildings in which we work and the required elements of the homes we go home to—is governed by rules and regulations. Not for nothing has the governance

framework for the entire US been referred to as "the modern administrative state."[53]

It is difficult to overstate the current significance of rules and regulations on our daily lives in the US (and, given federalism, each state also
enacts agency-driven rules and regulations). Agencies are remarkable
legal bodies in their own right. Although in virtually every instance agencies are creatures of the executive branch of government, in their affairs
they exercise powers belonging to all three branches of government. That
is, regulatory bodies draft and enact rules and regulations, they enforce
those enactments, and they adjudicate disputes arising under them.
Regulations therefore not only govern the daily lives of people in the US
to a large extent, but the agencies that govern pursuant to those regulations also have enormous influence over the affairs being regulated.

Regulatory capture is a critical part of the Manufacture of Doubt
and is widely regarded by legal and governance scholars as a form of
"government failure."[54] The problem arises in part because regulatory
bodies, almost by definition, must form relationships with the industries
whom they are regulating. The nature of the regulatory process, and
especially the rulemaking process, literally requires engagement with
the industry to be regulated. As chapter 4 will demonstrate, the deeper
these relationships go, the higher the likelihood of motivated bias and
behavior of partiality in favor of the industry. Essentially, when a regulatory body is captured by an industry, the agency tends to treat the
industry much more as a client to be served than a sophisticated commercial enterprise to be regulated at arms-length. This bias is visible in
virtually every significant case study that features the Manufacture of
Doubt.

In the case of silicosis, regulatory capture was especially apparent at
the National Silicosis Conference, a critical conference sponsored by the
Department of Labor that convened on April 14, 1936. Rosner and Markowitz explain that the industry action was coordinated by a key group
known as the Air Hygiene Foundation. Formed in 1935, the Air Hygiene
Foundation included representatives from virtually all of the so-called

dusty trades. The Foundation dominated the four committees at the conference, driving towards

> a consensus that would define the silicosis issue in the coming years and even decades. This consensus held that technologically feasible engineering and medical standards could be developed to prevent silicosis from shortening a person's worklife. The impact of silicosis was to be measured by its effect on a worker's ability to earn a living, not upon his or her own sense of well-being or the quality of his or her life after retirement.[55]

The Foundation's emphasis was on "business-dominated voluntary reform" and the workers' compensation system; "labor and its allies sought to move public policy . . . toward legislative and political efforts."[56] Moreover, as the Foundation developed, it increasingly began to mobilize medical and public health scientists into its service. First, it undertook an aggressive research program "that would become the basis for national voluntary standards in the field of occupational safety and health."[57] This program encouraged significant exchange and contact with leading scientists and physicians. Second, public health officials outright sympathized with the Air Hygiene Foundation. "Present and former officials in the Public Health Service and the Bureau of Mines, for example, moved easily between their public service in the US government and their private roles as employees and consultants to giant corporations and industrial trade associations."[58]

This particular issue is often referred to as the "revolving door problem," and it is a critical part of regulatory capture. The point for now is that prominent public health scientists, officials, and physicians were key players in the Foundation's efforts to manufacture doubt and sustain a regulatory vacuum. Indeed, Rosner and Markowitz note that "throughout the 1920s, companies had used physical examinations to discriminate against workers and had appropriated industrial physicians as 'company' doctors whose salary was paid by industry and whose loyalty was to those that paid them."[59] This quotation is important in demonstrating the strength of the framework in this book, since it obviously connects the railroad industry's conduct in the late nineteenth century to the Depression-era. In hiring physicians to manage risk and liability, the railroad industry began writing the script for the Manufacture of Doubt that industries would follow for the next 125 years to the present day. In Rosner and Markowitz's account, the various industries that exposed their workers to risks of silica and rock dust inhalation are displaying exactly the same behavior pioneered in important ways by the railroad industry almost 50 years earlier.

Nor is the phenomenon limited to the US. Australian environmental historian Jock McCulloch argues that many of the key components of the Manufacture of Doubt were developed by South African gold mine interests in the 1910s: "The gold mines can be seen as laboratories, which have paved the way for extractive industries to externalize their costs of production. That project began with the first Miners' Phthisis legislation, which outsourced the conduct of compensation medicals to the mining companies."[60] Note here again the use of internal, company-hired physician employees as an important feature in the Manufacture of Doubt. McCulloch points out that a great deal of the information we have regarding the conduct of the asbestos and tobacco industries in the US comes as a result of the discovery process required in US mass tort litigation (see chapter 6 for more on this critical issue). Because the South African gold mines were never subject to such litigation, the historical record of their conduct is comparatively sparse. Yet McCulloch notes one additional technique that the gold mining companies used to create doubt: they "swamp[ed] the public arena with misleading data. By 1925, the gold mines were collecting more than 100,000 dust samples a year. Because of the technologies used and the way the samples were averaged out to arrive at an abstract figure, such data could not identify specific hazards within individual mines."[61] We will see this technique again in the tobacco industry's use of the Manufacture of Doubt.

The Manufacture of Doubt is a social script that easily crosses political and national boundaries. Industries follow it because it works. It certainly "worked" in the silicosis case. Although two bills addressing silicosis originated in the Senate in the late 1930s, neither passed: "In context of the Depression and the oncoming mobilization for war, only the united support of the Roosevelt administration could have gotten the bill through Congress. In the closing months of the New Deal, the attention of the White House turned away from domestic legislation and toward preparation for war."[62]

The Public Health Service actually "opposed . . . the bill because it would strip it [the agency] of its authority over industrial disease."[63]After World War II, the issue became completely medicalized: "The views of labor and political reformers were no longer taken as seriously because the condition was now seen as the exclusive preserve of the scientific community. The language of science and medicine replaced the politics of negotiation in discussion of silicosis."[64] The legislative and political history of the battle over silicosis is complex and the details are beyond the scope of this book. Nevertheless, Rosner and Markowitz painstakingly document the variety of ways that the "dusty trades" collaborated to manufacture doubt, always working to forestall legislative and regulatory action. They would succeed in doing so until the early 1960s, when the US Congress passed a law that would guarantee Bureau of Mines inspectors the right of access. Nine years later, President Nixon signed into law a comprehensive workplace safety bill that, Rosner and Markowitz note, contained provisions first urged by the International Union of Mine, Mill, and Smelter Workers in 1956.[65]

In each of the two historical cases considered thus far, railroads and mines, we can see important components of the Manufacture of Doubt. These include but are not limited to

- employing company physicians and health professionals to review the injury/illness claims of workers and consumers;
- accusing injured/sick workers and/or consumers of malingering and feigning illness for the purposes of shoring up claims made in litigation;

- disputing causation between the product in question and adverse health;
- using anatomical evidence to undermine the injury/illness claims of workers and/or consumers;
- flooding the public arena with misleading or irrelevant data;
- hiring or partnering with public health officials, scientists, and physicians to conduct research, release press statements, and publish academic and scientific papers; and
- advancing regulatory capture.

Many of these strategies extend through other twentieth- and twenty-first-century applications of the Manufacture of Doubt and, as the analysis will show, some prove to be especially important. While many components of the Manufacture of Doubt are apparent in the case of the railroad industry and the "dusty trades," respiratory and circulatory health problems are also at the core of what is, without question, the single most successful industrial effort to manufacture doubt: the tobacco industry's campaign against the regulation of its products.

The Tobacco Industry and the Manufacture of Doubt

In this book, it is not possible to detail the tobacco industry's century-long program to manufacture doubt. Historians, public health scientists, and health care professionals have documented at length the incredible success that the tobacco industry enjoyed in developing what has been termed "agnotology"—the construction of ignorance.[66] While the tobacco industry did not invent many of the key techniques involved in the Manufacture of Doubt, they refined, developed, and extended them in far-reaching ways. As mentioned above, much of the information we have about the industry's behavior only came to light as a result of the public health litigation initiated largely by US states in the 1980s (private actors had attempted to sue the tobacco industry in tort for years, with mostly little success).

The very name of the social script stems in large part from an infamous 1969 internal memorandum sent from one marketing executive to another at the Brown & Williamson tobacco company:

> Doubt is our product since it is the best means of competing with the body of fact that exists in the mind of the general public. It is also the means of establishing that there is a controversy. If we are successful in establishing a controversy at the public level, then there is an opportunity to put across the real facts about smoking and health.[67]

"Doubt is our product." Historian of science Robert Proctor has provided a detailed list of the most influential strategies the tobacco industry used to manufacture doubt. These include:

- Publicize statements from scholars skeptical of the hazard.
- Publicize examples of people living to a ripe old age despite decades of smoking.
- Raise questions about "anomalies" that seem paradoxical: Why, if smoking causes cancer, do some countries with high rates of smoking have low rates of cancer?
- State that the evidence linking tobacco and disease is merely "statistical" and then deride statistics as an improper method for reasoning about causality.
- Put a positive spin on uncomfortable facts.
- Construct graphs and charts in such a way as to make it look like cancer trends are chaotic.
- Hire journalists to write industry-sympathetic articles in the popular press and pressure media organs to ignore or suppress reports unfavorable to industry.
- Undermine the authority of health organizations such as the American Cancer Society, the Surgeon General, the American Heart Association, or the National Cancer Institute.
- Hire historians to rewrite history from an industry point of view and then use such scholars as experts in courts.

- Proclaim the smoking and health controversy to be "nothing new," the "same old same old," and so forth.
- Keep people smoking by reassuring them that the industry is doing everything it can to make cigarettes as safe as possible and claim the high moral ground of corporate or environmental responsibility.[68]

Historian Allan Brandt charts the tobacco industry's ingenuity and fidelity to the program of agnotology. He argues that the emerging evidence that demonstrated a strong link between smoking and lung cancer rocked the industry to its foundations; the scope of the problem required the tobacco industry to undertake an entirely new strategy to ensure survival:

> They responded with a new and unprecedented public relations strategy. Its goal was to produce and sustain scientific skepticism and controversy in order to disrupt the emerging consensus on the harms of cigarette smoking. . . . The production of uncertainty in the face of the developing scientific knowledge required resources and skill. The industry worked to assure that vigorous debate would be prominently trumpeted in the public media. So long as there appeared to be doubt, so long as the industry could assert "not proven" . . . the industry would have cover to resist regulation of its product and the basis of a defense against new legal liabilities. The future of the cigarette would now depend on the successful production of a scientific controversy.[69]

The linchpin of the industry strategy began with a December 1953 meeting in the Plaza Hotel in New York City. There, Brandt notes, the CEOs of the major tobacco companies met and agreed to hire the prominent public relations firm of Hill & Knowlton. It was a fateful decision, one marked for its sagacity and correctness, at least when judged by the extent to which the tobacco industry achieved its objectives of manufacturing doubt and forestalling governance. Hill & Knowlton began by focusing on expanding partnerships with scientists and public health officials sympathetic to the industry and/or skeptical of the causal link between smoking and health. They urged the tobacco industry to abandon its past strategy of emphasizing the health benefits of individual brands. Instead, the industry "needed a collective research initiative to demonstrate its shared concern for the public."[70]

Mere weeks after being retained, Hill & Knowlton "had not only devised a major new strategic approach, but announced it to the media."[71] In early January 1954, they placed a major advertisement in "448 newspapers in 258 cities."[72] The advertisement announced the formation of the "Tobacco Industry Research Committee" and included text under the heading "A Frank Statement to Cigarette Smokers": "We accept an interest in people's health as a basic responsibility, paramount to every other consideration in this business. We believe the products we make are not injurious to health. We always have and always will cooperate closely with those whose task it is to safeguard the public health."[73]

Brandt observes that the so-called Frank Statement represented a true public relations triumph, almost single-handedly turning the tide of public opinion in favor of the tobacco industry: "The Frank Statement depicted an enlightened industry eager to fulfill its responsibilities to its patrons and the public. With obvious satisfaction, Hill & Knowlton staffers noted that editorials embraced the industry line as presented in the announcement."[74]

In his account, Proctor focuses especially on the extent to which the tobacco industry collaborated with academic scientists and scholars, including many historians. Such relationships are also present in many other cases in the Manufacture of Doubt, including in the silica and rock dust–producing industries and in the pharmaceutical industry. The next chapter analyzes the tackle football industry for signs of similar or overlapping strategies and techniques, but a specific strategy—connected to regulatory capture—was nearly perfected by the tobacco industry.

The type of regulatory capture practiced by the tobacco industry requires almost a complete switch in terminology from "regulatory" to "legislative." Regulators essentially had so little authority over the practices of the tobacco industry in the US (and in many other nation-states and regions of the globe), that there was little need for the industry to pursue capture. All of the "action" from a governance perspective occurred in the legislature and primarily in the US Congress (state governments only became involved in the latter decades of the twentieth century, and their efforts would eventually lead to the class-action litigation that marked the end, from a regulatory perspective, of what Brandt in 2007 famously termed "The Cigarette Century").

This lack of administrative law marks a critical issue in the overarching arguments of this book. If an industry succeeds in creating a regulatory vacuum that essentially eliminates all but the faintest trace of administrative governance, one might object that this shows that that industry is, in fact, unregulated. Chapter 3 analyzes this objection in more detail since it almost certainly applies to the tackle football industry (the NFL has been extremely successful in avoiding governance across the branches and sources of political authority).

For now, however, we can say that the objection confuses types with tokens. Whether a given industry manages to submit to or avoid regulation does not establish the criteria for the industry as a "regulated industry." Rather, that a particular industry has successfully mobilized social, political, and economic resources and strategies to achieve its ends (preventing governance) shows that in fact it is playing the political and social game of a "regulated industry." Congress finally granted the FDA authority over the tobacco industry in 2007; the industry had labored for decades to avoid this step—their efforts are primarily what prevented it from occurring much earlier. This illustrates the extent to which the tobacco industry had to "play the regulatory game." The industry's Manufacture of Doubt in actuality was such a game, one designed with a single paramount end: to escape the parameters of the game board itself. But it does not follow they were avoiding the regulatory game. They were not. They were playing it expertly.

In any event, the tobacco industry's tactics with Congress showed the basic hallmarks of a governance and advocacy strategy centered on the Manufacture of Doubt.[75] Peter D. Jacobsen and colleagues note that anti-smoking legislation (of any kind) "was not enacted until the second half of the 19th century, primarily in response to the fire hazard caused by smoking."[76] By the beginning of the twentieth century, "fourteen states had passed laws banning the production, sale, advertisement, or use of cigarettes within their boundaries. . . . As smoking grew in popularity, the laws were not enforced and, in many instances, were repealed."[77]

Jacobsen and colleagues argue that the record on federal activity governing tobacco is mixed. In 1938 Congress failed to define tobacco as a food or drug subject to FDA purview,[78] which dramatically limited administrative governance over tobacco until the 1960s at the absolute earliest. The surgeon general's landmark 1964 Report on Smoking and Health prompted Congress to act, mandating that warnings appear on all packages via the Federal Cigarette Labeling and Advertising Act of 1965. The Act expressly provided the Federal Trade Commission (FTC) with implementing power and preempted less stringent warnings under state law.

Faced with this regulatory fallout, the tobacco industry redesigned their product. They claimed that cigarettes could be made safer via the "low-tar" cigarette. Internal documents make clear that the tobacco industry knew full well that such cigarettes were, by almost any measure, no safer and in fact were potentially even more dangerous since smokers would take deeper, longer inhalations to ensure nicotine absorption.[79] But note this particular aspect in the Manufacture of Doubt: faced with increasing public and political pressure regarding the dangerousness of the product at the center of their commerce, the industry pivots to emphasize that the product can be made sufficiently safe. The tobacco industry is currently using exactly the same technique in its marketing strategies for e-cigarettes, arguing that the consumption of tobacco can be made sufficiently safe, ideally by the application of novel technologies.[80] Therefore, goes the argument, governance action is unwarranted, and whatever vacuum exists should persist, if not be expanded.

Following closely on the FTC's heels, the Federal Communications Commission (FCC) acquired governance authority over cigarette advertising under the 1969 Public Health Cigarette Smoking Act. The FTC subsequently entered into consent decrees with the tobacco industry in 1972 over the standardization of warning labels, followed by new legislation on labels in 1984, and bans on smoking on most domestic commercial airline flights in 1989.

Nevertheless, Jacobsen and colleagues are arguably too charitable. While federal legislative efforts were perceptible at various points in the twentieth century, the gaps between these points are long. The accumulation of days within these periods resulted in many millions of people suffering and dying. "Since 1964, when the U.S. Surgeon General warned that smoking caused cancer, the government estimates that tobacco has killed more than 20 million Americans. That is 15 times the number of Americans who have perished in all wars combined."[81] This general idea is crucial and forms the bulk of the analysis in chapter 6: public health laws must be understood as social determinants of health in their own right. The laws and policies a given polity enacts, or chooses not to enact, have an enormous influence on the particular distribution of health in that population. Thus, while federal governance of tobacco has been more than zero, there is nevertheless consensus that the extent and scope of that governance is spotty at best until the 1990s. This public health law vacuum had utterly devastating health consequences in the US.

Moreover, given the advent of both state and federal regulatory action in the early 1990s, one would predict that the tobacco industry would deploy some of the same strategies intended to facilitate regulatory capture. Recall that because Congress had never specifically declared tobacco a "drug" under the 1938 Food, Drug and Cosmetic Act, the FDA essentially had never behaved as if it had regulatory authority over the tobacco industry. However, given the changing legal landscapes wrought by mass tort litigation at the end of the 1980s, the FDA commissioner during the mid-1990s, David Kessler, expressly sought to assert regulatory authority over the tobacco industry. David Nye documents that this possibility triggered a range of anxieties for the tobacco industry: on the table could be anything from

> concerns about prohibitions on the sale of tobacco products to issues related to advertising bans, prescribing tar and nicotine yields on a brand-by-brand basis, limiting the use of additives, requiring full disclosure of additives on pack labels, requiring strong and prominent pack label warnings, and the power of the FDA to conduct factory inspections and access company documents on manufacturing processes.[82]

Under the Clinton Administration, the FDA declared regulatory authority over the tobacco industry in August 1996. The ensuing litigation concluded only at the US Supreme Court in 2000, resulting in a narrow 5–4 decision against the FDA.[83] Congress itself would have to intervene, specifically granting the FDA authority over the tobacco industry in the 2009 Family Smoking Prevention and Tobacco Control Act.[84]

The extensive history of the tobacco industry's Manufacture of Doubt is an immense literature, one that is literally still growing daily (as millions of pages of tobacco industry documents can be mined with sophisticated algorithmic search techniques to show all sorts of interesting and significant findings). But one specific technique, so expertly honed by the tobacco industry, is at the very core of the Manufacture of Doubt currently at work in the American tackle football industry: sowing doubt as to causation.

Causation and Doubt

During the middle decades of the twentieth century, the tobacco industry's central problem became increasingly clear. The rapidly accumulating evidence pointed to a strong link between smoking tobacco products and severe adverse health outcomes. Although the tobacco industry treated these links matter-of-factly by the late 1950s,[85] they understood that the causal inference Americans were increasingly willing to draw, in connecting smoking to ill health (and lung cancer in particular), was hugely problematic both for the profitability of their enterprise and for the always-looming specter of regulatory authority. The more that the public and key political figures believed that tobacco posed a serious public health problem, the more likely the industry was to face governance and regulation.

Challenging the causal links between exposure to the company's product and the injured consumer is not new to the tobacco industry. The analysis above shows that the railroad industry engaged in exactly this activity, practically sponsoring an entire field of health care (railway medicine and surgery) in part for the purpose of undermining causal claims between a railway accident and an ensuing injury. The railroad industry relied in part on claims to scientific and medical objectivity generated from anatomical, photographic, and, later, radiographic evidence. As noted above, the silica and rock dust–producing industries did the same, with an increased emphasis on X-rays as the medium for discerning the alleged truth of the matter.

Thus, challenging the evidence for the causal link between exposure and public health harm is at the core of the Manufacture of Doubt. It is original, in an important sense. Moreover, such challenging is both a key strategy and a goal in itself. Generating doubt as to the causal links between the exposure and the harm is a political strategy and an important industrial product (literally—"doubt is our product," as a tobacco company executive stated). While the tobacco industry did not invent this technique, they refined and made expert use of it. Proctor documents how as late as 1960, an American Cancer Society poll showed that "only a third of all US doctors agreed that cigarette smoking should be considered 'a major cause of lung cancer.'"[86] The tobacco industry "spent countless sums to deny and distract from the cigarette-cancer link, in some instances actually quantifying the impact of their denialist propaganda."[87]

Proctor explains that in 1972, the tobacco industry hired a market research firm to assess the impact of its propaganda film, "Smoking and Health: The Need to Know."

> Prior to screening viewers were asked a series of questions about whether the Surgeon General "could be wrong about the dangers of smoking"; the same questions were then asked after the screening. . . . [T]he Tobacco Institute was happy to report that the film had reduced the number of people agreeing that "Cigarette smoking cause[s] lung cancer" by 17.8% (from 74.9% to 57.1%). The film had also produced "significant shifts" in attitudes favourable to the industry in other areas, including whether recent reports had "overemphasized the dangers of smoking."[88]

Chapter 5 goes into much more detail explaining why the question of causation is so ripe for attack using the Manufacture of Doubt, and what can be done about it. Proving that a given exposure causes a particular health outcome is often difficult in complex epidemiologic contexts. Regulated industries have consistently preferred to seize on that difficulty in gaining a foothold to construct ignorance.

Yussuf Saloojee and Elif Dagli note that, despite virtual consensus within the tobacco industry by the late 1950s that smoking causes lung cancer, smoking advertisements continued to deny causation, as in this 1969 example for Brown & Williamson:

> Ten years ago there was a cancer scare over the wax in milk cartons. And over using iodine to get a suntan. These theories were about as valid as the one that says toads cause warts. And they're about as valid as today's scare tactics surrounding cigarettes. Because no one has been able to produce conclusive proof that cigarette smoking causes cancer. Scientific, biological, clinical, or any other kind.[89]

Note the use of the phrase "conclusive proof"; the industry need not deny the existence of any kind of correlation between the product and the health harm. Even by the 1960s that kind of outright denial strained what little credibility the tobacco industry enjoyed; the strategy is simply to sow doubt, to argue that the connections are not conclusively proven, that further scientific research is required.

During over four decades of almost completely successful mass tort litigation, many hundreds of expert medical and scientific witnesses repeatedly testified for the tobacco industry in ways that cast doubt on causation. In 2006 a detailed study that harvested data from the Tobacco Deposition and Trial Testimony Archive (DATTA) project (a result of the tobacco litigation itself), Sharon Milberger and colleagues found that the industry argued that there is no proof smoking causes lung cancer in a preponderance of its tort defense between 1986 and 2003.[90] The authors also found that the tobacco industry's use of the anti-causation argument declined from 89% of cases before 1997 to only 25% of cases in 2003.[91] Nevertheless, one study of otolaryngologists who testified on behalf of the tobacco industry between 2009 and 2014 indicated that such efforts to deny causation endures virtually to the present. Indeed, while the landmark tobacco litigation settlements required the industry to admit causation, the industry continues to deny it in individual legal cases:

> This tactical approach is abetted by legions of well-compensated "experts," who provide testimony proffering alternative causations for smokers who develop cancers of types typically caused by tobacco. Tobacco legal defense teams have honed methods to implant the notion in the jury that tobacco's role in a plaintiff's cancer is controversial and that the scientific evidence is debatable. Their strategy is to manufacture doubt in the mind of jurors, who lack the technical background needed to critically analyze testimony on cancer causation.[92]

Milberger and colleagues note that some public statements of individual tobacco corporations "accept general causality while rejecting individual causality."[93] This means that even while some companies admitted that in general smoking causes lung cancer, "we know of no way to verify that smoking is a cause of any particular person's adverse health or why smoking may have adverse health effects on some people and not others."[94]

×××

The vast scope of industrial activity in scripting and enacting the Manufacture of Doubt in the twentieth and early twenty-first century is literally the subject of thousands of scholarly and popular works. Major actors in this space, such as the automobile, commercial airplane, and pharmaceutical industries have barely been mentioned. The preceding analysis has sketched just a small part of the historical arc that the Manufacture of Doubt has taken in US history. Specifically, this chapter focused on several case studies of considerable importance in developing, practicing, and refining the script as a way of tracing just a few of its key features. The analysis here cannot cover the full spectrum of attitudes, practices, beliefs, and tactics that constitute the script.

Nevertheless, the discussion here describes many of the most historically, legally, and politically significant elements of the Manufacture of Doubt. The question now is the extent to which these elements apply to the US tackle football industry and its behavior. Chapter 3 undertakes the task of answering that question.

The American Tackle Football Industry's Manufacture of Doubt

In this chapter, the analysis proceeds by considering squarely the question of whether American tackle football is fairly deemed a regulated industry. If it is not, many of the arguments advanced in the remainder of this book will likely be unpersuasive. Indeed, if American tackle football does not qualify as a regulated industry, it is unclear how and why the Manufacture of Doubt would be a particularly useful script to follow. Recall that social scripts are inextricably linked to their impact on human behavior; the concept originates primarily in the field of social psychology. Behavior is highly context-specific; if American tackle football does not unfold in the context of a regulated industry, it is not obvious why the behaviors normed by the Manufacture of Doubt would be useful or even appropriate.

Thus, the first question is whether American tackle football is fairly regarded as a regulated industry. An affirmative answer leads to the second question: whether some of the most prominent techniques used in the Manufacture of Doubt are evident amidst the political, legal, and social contests over collision sports, TBI, and injury.

Is American Tackle Football a Regulated Industry?

Whether American tackle football can be regarded as a regulated industry has profound public health implications and grave ethical significance. The public health implications flow from the idea that laws, or their absence, ought to be regarded as an independent social determinant of health. There is strong evidence for this idea. This implies that law ought to be regarded as an epidemiologic exposure, analogous to any other exposure and studied as objects of scientific and epidemiologic analysis. In fact, this is exactly a central claim of chapter 6. The nascent fields of legal epidemiology and public health law research have arisen to ask questions along the lines noted here (to discern where and how law determines health outcomes).

There are also normative ethical implications that flow from the impact of governance on population health. If American tackle football is a regulated industry, then it falls under the purview of a governance structure that can reach both wide and deep to administer the ways the product is marketed, distributed, and sold. Regulatory bodies can compel corporations to alter the structure of their labor arrangements. Indeed, this is exactly what an interdisciplinary team of researchers connected to the Petrie-Flom Center for Health Law Policy, Biotechnology, and Bioethics at Harvard Law School urged. In 2018, three law professors joined a practicing attorney litigating cases against the NFL and an environmental health scholar to argue that federal occupational health and safety laws should apply to the NFL.[1] (Such laws have generally not been implemented or enforced with regard to professional tackle football.)

Chapter 4 will evaluate this specific proposal in some detail; the important point for now is the question, and the increasing tendency among all manner of stakeholders, to regard American tackle football as a regulated industry. Some scholars might object to this characterization on the grounds that American tackle football has largely escaped significant federal and state regulation. Indeed, the NFL, like other professional sports leagues, has obtained an antitrust exemption from the US Congress, which means that the ability to use a sphere of law to govern the NFL has specifically been eliminated by an act of Congress.

Nevertheless, this objection is only superficially plausible and falls apart under closer inspection. Initially, the term "regulated industry" cannot be taken literally. Although its meaning is not limited to the legal domain, from a public health law standpoint, the phrase does not imply anything at all regarding the scope of the regulation governing the industry. Rather, it is a legal term-of-art that creates a juridical category (industries that are subject to regulatory purview even if the powers themselves are rarely exercised).

Not unique among sophisticated industries, the NFL has been remarkably successful in avoiding governance and regulation. Concluding that the NFL and its partners are not drivers of a regulated industry is invalid in the technical sense because the conclusion is not implied directly from the premise. That is, it is possible that the NFL has been successful in avoiding governance and regulation and that the NFL is a regulated industry. And, in fact, this is correct. The proof for this is in the very idea of the Manufacture of Doubt as a social script.

Regulated industries deploy the Manufacture of Doubt because it works. The script is a way of anticipating, as well as reacting to, efforts to use the machinery of regulation and the administrative state to govern the commerce of the industry. Actors who use the Manufacture of Doubt uniformly do so as a way of managing the risk of governance, the threat of which stems primarily from regulatory sources. Pressing the script into successful service fails to imply that the industry in question is not regulated; rather it shows that the industry has executed a complex legal and political strategy that results in its continual escape from the arms of the regulatory state. In other words, case studies which demonstrate highly successful use of the Manufacture of Doubt also prove a central claim of this book: the relevant example is a regulated industry. Its success in avoiding regulation is a point in favor of the claim.[2]

If there were any further doubts regarding the merits of American tackle football as a regulated industry, consider the exact words of Jon Butler, the executive director of Pop Warner, which is the governing body for youth football in the US and which has strong ties with the NFL. In a 2019 article published online at CBS Sports, Butler stated: "First, we have a duty to football. This means too much to people and has for so long we can't turn our back on it. We figured out tobacco. We figured out asbestos. We'll figure this out."[3]

This quote is astonishing. Leaving aside for the moment the questions of whether anyone owes a moral duty to "football," and if so who specifically owes such a duty, consider that the North American leader of youth football in 2019 explicitly lists the sport in an analogical series with tobacco and asbestos. Moreover, who is the "we" that "figured out" tobacco and asbestos? It is not the tackle football industry, which Butler helps lead, since it is absurd to say that the football industry "figured out" tobacco and asbestos. Rather, the more plausible inference is that Butler sees himself and his fellow leaders in the football industry as part of a tradition of industrialists who grapple with political and legal forces seeking to curb the harmful exposures associated with use of the relevant products. If this is correct, then it is not only the case that the national leader of youth football in the US in 2019 thinks that football is a regulated industry that is injurious to public health. Apparently, said leader also sees as a current objective for the football industry the attempt to "figure out" ways to minimize—presumably—the legal and regulatory efforts to provide effective governance over the harmful product.

Furthermore, the claim that the tobacco and asbestos industries "figure[d] [it] out" seems either incoherent or absurd. What does it mean to say that the industries "figured out" a problem that was associated with extensive injury, illness, and death from the use of their respective products? To the extent this claim is meant to assert that both industries resolved their problems with tort litigation in a manner comporting with basic mandates of justice, it is extremely dubious (see chapter 6). The historical record for both tobacco and asbestos incontrovertibly shows that both industries were extremely active and effective utilizers of the Manufacture of Doubt. Their success resulted in decades of additional health harms to end-users.

American tackle football is unquestionably a regulated industry. The next question is whether the tackle football industry manufactures doubt.

American Tackle Football and the Manufacture of Doubt: A Family Resemblance Analysis

The Manufacture of Doubt is a social script. Although such scripts normalize behavior, they are also shaped and molded by the various actions that the relevant actors take. Recall from chapter 1 that social scripts are not fate. Individuals and groups maintain some agency and can react to complex motivations and interests in unpredictable ways. Moreover, actors create new ways to manufacture doubt, ways not established in earlier iterations of the script. Those ways in turn become synthesized into the next iterations of the script, in a basic dialectic.

Why does any of this matter? One reason is because to define the Manufacture of Doubt in terms of strict criteria makes little sense. Any given actor may use all, some, or even none of the generally established techniques deployed to construct ignorance. In the latter case, for strategic policy reasons, an actor may stay relatively inactive for a period of time, discerning that it is not in their current political interests to engage processes of public reason and to attempt robustly to manufacture doubt in the public sphere. Furthermore, as noted, actors may create new techniques to manufacture doubt, which by definition cannot be previously established criteria. Thus, trying to define the Manufacture of Doubt in terms of criteria that must be necessary and sufficient to produce the scripted behavior is inadvisable or even incoherent.

We want to define the Manufacture of Doubt because we need to know whether, and the extent to which, it may apply to the actions of any given regulated industry. If we don't have a clear picture of the concept, we simply won't be able to form a well-reasoned opinion about whether, say, the American tackle football industry's behavior is an instance of the Manufacture of Doubt.

Thus, we require a method to define the Manufacture of Doubt that does not rely on strict criteria. Fortunately, we have the needed conceptual apparatus to do so: philosopher Ludwig Wittgenstein's idea of family resemblances. As I have argued elsewhere:

> The appeal to Wittgenstein is justified here because the conception of meaning Wittgenstein articulated in his later career specifically rejects the need to delineate necessary and sufficient conditions for a word or concept in order for it to have meaning. That is, Wittgenstein argued precisely that we use words and phrases in practice quite meaningfully without needing or possessing definitions for that language. Specifically, Wittgenstein articulated the idea of *family resemblances* in explicating the idea of a game. He denied that speakers require the existence of an essence, of any core feature of what makes a game of chess, for example, different from a game of backgammon, in order to speak of these games meaningfully.[4]

The point is simply that we can understand the Manufacture of Doubt absent any reliance on strict criteria. The behaviors and techniques that comprise the script are both meaningful and sensible to its participants as well as to outside observers in terms of these family resemblances. These family resemblances have also been conceptualized as "X-making characteristics," where X equals the particular language game in which we are playing and/or are interested.

> In place of the notion of a necessary and sufficient condition that corresponds to each individual word, Wittgenstein argued for the notion of family resemblances, of a kind of malleable similarity that serves to connect particular uses of the same word. As one commentator puts it, Wittgenstein's idea is that a family is not a family because they resemble one another but that because they resemble one another they exist as a family. . . . [U]nder Wittgenstein's analysis, we can play a given language game quite meaningfully even if there is no necessary and sufficient condition that satisfies all instances of a word's usage.[5]

Accordingly, there is no need to attempt to define the Manufacture of Doubt based on traditional ideas of necessary and sufficient criteria.

It is in fact either impossible or inadvisable. We can, however, under-stand key aspects of the Manufacture of Doubt in terms of family re-semblances, key components of the language game that help make the Manufacture of Doubt cohere as a family. Chapter 2 has already detailed a number of these key "Manufacture-of-Doubt-making-characteristics." These characteristics are summarized in table 1 across the industries explicitly considered thus far, along with three other regulated indus-tries (the pharmaceutical, lead, and food industries) and American tackle football.

The single question remaining in this chapter is whether American tackle football, as a regulated industry, has mobilized any of these tech-niques in the Manufacture of Doubt. The answer is simple: yes. The American tackle football industry has in fact used almost all of the script-making characteristics listed in table 1. We'll look at each of these char-acteristics below. (Note that the characteristic "advancing regulatory capture" is not discussed below; the extensive use of regulatory capture by the tackle football industry is a primary theme of this book and is discussed extensively in chapters 2, 4, and 6.)

Manufacture doubt by employing company health
care providers
The first characteristic under consideration here is the employ-ment of company physicians and health professionals to review the illness/injury claims of workers and/or consumers. In the NFL, health care professionals are hired directly by each individual team—each team is an independent business organization—to diagnose, remedy, and ultimately provide health care services for the players. The conflicts of interest here are so manifest they have generated scholarly opprobrium since the 1970s. There is abundant evidence to conclude that this ar-rangement has not generally produced results consistent with the best interests of the players.[6]

Virtually every other major regulated industry—perhaps virtually every large employer—in the US has largely abandoned the model of

Table 1. Key script-making characteristics of the Manufacture of Doubt used by different industries

Script-Making Characteristic	Railroad	Dust/Mining	Tobacco	Pharmaceutical	Lead	Food	American Tackle Football
Employing company physicians and health professionals to review the injury/illness claims of workers and consumers	Yes	Yes	No	Yes	Yes	No	Yes
Accusing injured/sick workers and/or consumers of malingering and feigning illness for the purposes of shoring up claims made in litigation	Yes	Yes	Yes	Yes	Yes	No	Yes
Disputing causation between the product in question and adverse health	Yes	Yes	Yes	Yes	Yes	Yes	Yes
Using anatomical evidence to undermine the injury/illness claims of workers and consumers	Yes	Yes	Yes	Yes	Yes	No	Yes
Flooding the public arena with misleading or irrelevant data	Yes	Yes	Yes	Yes	Yes	Yes	Yes
Hiring or partnering with public health officials, scientists, and physicians to conduct research, release press statements, and publish academic and scientific papers	Yes	Yes	Yes	Yes	Yes	Yes	Yes
Advancing regulatory capture	Yes	Yes	Yes	Yes	Yes	Yes	Yes
Claiming to design and sell a significantly "safer" version of the product in question	Yes	Yes	Yes	Yes	Yes	Yes	Yes

direct care provided by employer-salaried providers. The NFL is the only multibillion-dollar industry remaining that embraces this model of care. Chapter 4 will take up these matters in detail, but for now it is worth noting that this model of care is the very same one pioneered by the railroad industry. And, just as with the railroad industry, there is no question that the NFL team physicians have, for at least four decades, been embroiled in the processes of tort litigation. Indeed, over that time period, NFL team physicians have been involved in virtually every component of tort litigation brought against the NFL, in both individual and class suits.

Moreover, it is wrong to think only in terms of actual litigation (i.e., marked by the filing of a pleading or a demand letter). Tort litigation is a liability assessment system, one that legal scholars agree is frequently intertwined with questions of policy.[7] The model of care the NFL relies on for its workers is one that as a policy matter compels team physicians and health care providers to think constantly about the liability to which their employer is exposed by the hazardous product being marketed. This is exactly what happened with health care professionals directly employed by the railroad industry.

Legal scholars and ethicists are virtually united in their insistence that this model of care is morally untenable and should be abandoned; a team of investigators at Harvard Law School released a lengthy report in 2018 where they strongly endorsed a move away from this model of care and provided detailed analysis and evidence in support of the recommendation.[8] While the details of this will be addressed in the next chapter, the point here is that the first "script-making characteristic" is at work in the American tackle football industry. It should also be noted that tackle football teams at many different levels (college, high school, and increasingly even younger leagues and associations) sponsor team health care professionals—often athletic trainers—to provide care directly to players. While college football players are involved in increasing legal efforts to establish their status as workers, no one yet regards high school or younger-aged participants as workers. Nevertheless, the idea that teams should directly employ health care professionals to tend to the injuries and illnesses of their players is one that permeates much of the American tackle football industry. This is unsurprising given the wide consensus that the behavior of the NFL and its constituent teams has an enormous impact in shaping tackle football culture and norms "downstream" among the millions of youths and adolescents that play the game.

The conclusion is obvious: The American tackle football industry has earnestly practiced this first technique in the Manufacture of Doubt.

Manufacture doubt by accusing injured/sick workers
and/or consumers of "malingering"

The second script-making characteristic is accusing sick or injured workers and/or consumers of malingering or feigning illness.[9] Regulated industries embroiled in tort litigation often deploy this strategy, as the connections between anxieties over such litigation and accusations of malingering are at least as old as the railroad industry. Both the NFL as a corporate entity and many of its coaches have voiced such accusations against its players—the primary workforce.

For example, in 2014, journalist Patrick Hruby, who has tirelessly analyzed the TBI problem in the NFL, turned his critical eye to the settlement agreement effectively ending the first round of class action TBI litigation against the league. He noted that the agreement itself seemed to encourage easy accusations of malingering. Specifically, the agreement provided that former players seeking recovery must submit to neuropsychological testing. "To weed out people who are attempting to fake brain injuries, neuropsychological testers use a concept called 'malingering.' Over a series of exams, sometimes lasting as long as five hours, patients are expected to give a consistent, emotionally-neutral effort—if they don't, there's a good chance they'll be labeled as frauds."[10]

The problem, as Hruby notes, is that many former players experience physical and emotional impairments, including pain and all manner of mental illness. They are as a class extremely unlikely to be able to sit still for the required five hours, increasing the chances that the testing will suggest "malingering." Or consider journalist Andrew Heisel's 2014 account of the case of Joe McCall.[11] In 1986, McCall played for the (NFL) Tampa Bay Buccaneers, and he was suffering from a knee injury that rendered him unable to play. Then-operative league rules left the team responsible for McCall's salary until he was cleared to play. The team therefore had a vested interest in proving that "he wasn't injured, that he was a faker, a malinger."[12] At a visit with team doctors for therapy on his knee, the doctors injected him with sodium pentathol—the unreliable "truth serum" widely used by law enforcement and the Central Intelligence Agency. Their intent was obvious, as McCall recalled experiencing the equivalent of an "inquisition." Later, one of the doctors present admitted to both the objective and the use of the sodium pentathol, and blamed it on a since-retired physician on the team.[13]

While the Joe McCall story is extreme, the NFL's interest in undermining the illness and injury claims of its workers through accusations of malingering is a common enough theme. It is, for example, rampant in the history of the NFL's disability and benefit determination scheme, which in both structure and practice systematically disenfranchised and diminished the scope of pension benefits available to retired players. Many of the plaintiffs in the ensuing pension litigation were poor or struggling—some had played in an era where the salaries were relatively modest and were now being crushed by the weight of significant chronic illnesses, lack of wealth or earning power, and in at least some cases, dementia, CTE, or other serious neuropathologies. In a series of successes that should evoke the tobacco industry's work in this area, the NFL unerringly prevailed in both administrative appeals and resulting litigation. The NFL won so much that in 2005, when a federal district court reversed a determination of the NFL's Disability Board, it prompted the completion of an entire law review article to mark the occasion. The article is "One for Twenty-Five: The Federal Courts Reverse a Decision of the NFL's Disability Board for the First Time since 1993 in *Jani v. Bert Bell/Pete Rozelle NFL Player Retirement Plan*."[14]

In 2012 a group of experts published an anthology titled *Detection of Malingering during Head Injury Litigation*.[15] There is no evidence that the editors have close relationships with the tackle football industry. Nevertheless, the anthology is transparently targeted at professionals serving or intending to serve as expert witnesses in head injury litigation. The use of such experts is most certainly part of the Manufacture of Doubt—indeed, tort litigation is itself wielded as an artifact to construct doubt in the public sphere (see table 1).

Moreover, there is a history of NFL coaches accusing injured players of malingering. Former coach Tom Coughlin was notorious for mocking and belittling his injured players, referring to them derisively as the "sick, lame, and lazy."[16] Former player Ted Johnson has publicly indicated that he lives with Second Impact Syndrome, throbbing headaches, and significant mood problems. In 2009 he stated that his coach had pressured him to participate in full contact drills three days after experiencing a first concussion. He experienced a second concussion during the drills, an especially dangerous event capable of causing sudden massive brain injury, although it did not occur in this case.

In short, there is ample evidence that the NFL, its representatives, and supervisors in positions of authority over players (i.e., coaches) have accused workers of feigning illness, faking, and/or malingering.

Manufacture doubt by disputing causation between the product and adverse health

This script-making characteristic is so significant in the history of the American tackle football industry's efforts to manufacture doubt, it is practically emblematic of the entire campaign. The NFL in particular has made challenging causation the centerpiece of its agnotological efforts (that is, its efforts to construct ignorance), and with good reason: the NFL obviously learned from the tobacco industry's sharp, enduring success in crafting regulatory capture and constructing ignorance through the use of this particular technique.

Although there are many excellent sources and accounts of the NFL's efforts to deny causation, perhaps they are most well-curated in the 2013 documentary *League of Denial*.[17] Sponsored by the ESPN sports television network, brothers and investigative journalists Mark Fainaru-Wada and Steve Fainaru laid out in excruciating detail the NFL's decades-long effort to manufacture doubt regarding the connection between playing football and long-term neuropathology, especially CTE. Scandal shrouded even the release of the documentary. PBS, the producer of the documentary through its award-winning program *Frontline*, announced a release date of October 8, 2013. On August 23, 2013, the *New York Times* ran a front-page article that addressed ESPN's stunning decision to withdraw its sponsorship of the documentary less than three months before it premiered.[18]

ESPN faced a terrible conflict of interest in sponsoring the documentary; it enjoyed a multibillion dollar contract with the NFL to broadcast its games. Sponsoring a documentary squarely positioning the NFL among the ranks of despised health-harming industries such as tobacco would hardly benefit ESPN's extremely lucrative relationship with the league. So, while few were truly shocked by ESPN's decision to withdraw official sponsorship of the documentary, the *Times* article contained details of a certain lunch meeting between extremely high-level officials representing ESPN and the NFL, held at a midtown Manhattan restaurant named Patroon. Four people attended this lunch: NFL Commissioner Roger Goodell (the equivalent of the CEO of the league), president of the NFL Network Steve Bornstein, ESPN President John Skipper, and ESPN's executive vice-president for production John Wildhack.[19] "The meeting was combative, the people said, with league officials conveying their irritation with the direction of the documentary, which is expected to describe a narrative that has been captured in various news reports over the past decade: the league turning a blind eye to evidence that players were sustaining brain trauma on the field that could lead to profound, long-term cognitive disability."[20]

ESPN denied that the NFL had requested it withdraw its sponsorship and claimed it had done so out of a dispute over editorial control of the film. But, as the article noted, ESPN's "dual mandate" to report objectively on the NFL and broadcast its games as a financial and television partner, meant that "few direct requests would have had to have been made."[21]

In any event, both the documentary and the ensuing book detail the lengths to which the tackle football industry has gone to dispute the causal connections between exposure and adverse health outcomes.[22] The details are innumerable.

For example, consider the case of Elliot Pellman, the long-time chair of the NFL's Traumatic Brain Injury Committee (NFL-TBIC). The NFL-TBIC itself has a significant history, some of which was the subject of interrogation during congressional hearings in 2009 and 2010. In October 2006, *ESPN The Magazine* published a detailed report on the NFL-TBIC, listing numerous troubling features.[23] "First, the NFL-TBIC had steadfastly refused to accept any of the reported findings of links between mild TBI and long-term TBI, insisting that it was safe for NFL players to return to full-contact action on the same day that they suffered the concussion. . . . Second, Pellman, the long-time chair of the NFL-TBIC, is a rheumatologist by training with no expertise in neurology."[24]

Third, there was evidence that the NFL had sponsored a research study, with Pellman as principal investigator, that simply neglected to include data from hundreds of current players.[25] During the time Pellman chaired the NFL-TBIC, the NFL steadfastly and almost without exception denied the existence of a causal link between playing professional tackle football and neuropathology. Pellman also served as lead author on a number of publications, which we'll discuss below.

At the 2009 congressional hearings, former NFL player Bernie Parrish, who was for a time lead plaintiff in a class action suit filed against the NFL and the NFL Players Association (NFLPA) over lost licensing and royalty fees, had this to say:

> This mild traumatic brain injury committee is the sequel to the tobacco council which produced its own bogus studies, paid experts to testify that

tobacco products do not cause cancer, and it exactly parallels the way that Covington & Burling partner Paul Tagliabue, who was commissioner of the NFL, set up and created the NFL's Mild Traumatic [Brain] Injury Committee. He named the first chairman, Elliott Pellman, who was his personal physician and a graduate of Guadalajara's Medical School in Rheumatology, who had absolutely no expertise on brain injuries. . . .

. . . [S]o we're, you know, we're kind of—keep going back to square one, and I keep going back—it takes me right back to the tobacco industry, the way they sold the fact that using tobacco products doesn't cause cancer, playing professional football doesn't cause dementia eventually, etcetera. And the idea that the—they have perfected deny—the delay and deny process, delay, delay, study it, study it to death, and make magnanimous statements about what they're going to do, etcetera, etcetera, wind up denying.[26]

Peering a little deeper into the rhetoric of NFL Commissioner Roger Goodell at the 2009 hearings reveals more regarding this absolutely critical characteristic of the Manufacture of Doubt—and the tackle football industry's embrace of it. Goodell, it should be mentioned, is Tagliabue's hand-picked successor and is still reigning commissioner. Though he is careful in his remarks, one can, with little difficulty, discern subtle attempts to manufacture doubt.

In his prepared comments, Goodell testified: "We know that concussions are a serious matter, and that they will require special attention and treatment. And in this area, I have been clear. Medical considerations must always come first."[27] This is an entirely reasonable statement; so reasonable, in fact, that there is virtually nothing with which to take exception. However, the rub is in the vagueness of the phrase "medical considerations." The definition of medical considerations that come first is left wide open, as is the criteria of action that constitutes the extension of "comes first." And again, the apparent reasonableness of the questions and statements by leading industry officials is a hallmark of the manufacture of doubt strategies. Blanket denials are simply not credible and must therefore be wrapped in a package of accommodation and reasonableness. As the hearing reveals, the nature of such strategies is not lost on all of the participants.

Goodell's prepared testimony is consistent with rhetoric and techniques past actors accused of industrial harm have deployed. Several of the participants in the 2009 hearing demonstrate awareness of such tactics and attempt to pin down the commissioner. Thus, Representative John Conyers (a Democrat from Michigan) uses some of his allotted time to ask Goodell directly: "Is there a link between playing professional football and the likelihood of contracting a brain-related injury such as dementia, Alzheimer's, depression, or CTE?"[28] Goodell's response exemplifies the Manufacture of Doubt: "You are obviously seeing a lot of data and a lot of information that our committees and others have presented, with respect to the linkage. And the medical experts should be the one to be able to continue that debate."[29] Goodell claims ignorance, frames the question as a purely scientific and medical one for which only those with the requisite technical expertise should be permitted to opine, and suggests the pressing question—of whether the kinds of injuries that are common in American football are a causal factor in serious and long-term neuropathology—remains in question.

Goodell hastens to add that "we are not waiting for that debate to continue," thereby emphasizing, again, the NFL's accommodationist vantage point even on issues of great uncertainty. Goodell is undoubtedly aware of both the need to appear flexible and reasonable. Representative Conyers, however, is not interested in Goodell's evasion: "I just asked you a simple question. What is the answer?"[30] Goodell will not capitulate: "The answer is, the medical experts would know better than I would with respect to that."[31]

In the hearing, Goodell consistently stuck to the program of establishing doubt and uncertainty. In response to a question asking about future steps, Goodell asserts that "the first thing we have to do is continue to support this research and make sure we put more and more into this research so that we can find out what exactly are the medical facts."[32]

This statement implies, first, that the medical facts regarding causal links between exposure and adverse health outcomes remain in doubt, and, second, that the top priority should be further research on the extent of such causal links. The latter is both entirely reasonable—who would oppose attempts to advance scientific knowledge on the subject?—and is also dilatory because it implies that absent further findings it would be premature to act on the basis that any such causal link exists. This connection between the denial of causation and a preferred policy (inaction—the vacuum) is hugely important and is a central subject of chapter 5. Goodell's statement here also ignores the fact that the NFL's pre-2009 sponsored research on the long-term health implications of TBI were almost universally panned as being shoddy and pervaded by extensive conflicts of interest (the subject of the following chapter).

Representative Conyers was not alone in his skepticism of Goodell's attempts to manufacture doubt. Representative Anthony Weiner (a Democrat from New York), himself a former college football player, noted the NFL's history of obfuscation and denials regarding the links between TBI and serious brain disease, at one point reminding Goodell that "the NFL has said research has not shown any long-term problems in NFL players. I mean obviously that is—I mean today I doubt you would say that multiple concussions don't create long-term problems today knowing what you do now."[33] Goodell's response: "Well, we want Congress, we want the medical community, we want everyone involved to have confidence in the work that is being done, and that is why we have medical professionals involved. That is why we put it up for peer review and why they choose that."[34] This too is a non sequitur that evades Representative Weiner's question entirely, and again advances the claim that the task of determining the state of the risk is one best left to the physicians and scientists alone.

On the merits, Goodell's claim is mistaken for a variety of reasons, not least because the assessment of risk from a public health perspective unquestionably involves normative judgments. While good science and epidemiology may help calibrate the risk, the question of what levels of risk are acceptable for which populations are unavoidably moral and political questions, which, as I have noted, must be resolved politically if they are to be resolved at all. As Kerianne H. Quanstrum and Rodney A. Heyward put it, "Scientific evidence can only help us describe the continuum of benefit versus harm. The assessment of whether the benefit is great enough to warrant the risk of harm—i.e., the decision of where the threshold for intervention should lie—is necessarily a value judgment."[35] I have labeled this aspect of public health policymaking the "unbearable oughtness of public health policy," and therefore Goodell is quite wrong in suggesting that the task of assessing acceptable levels of risk is one reserved for physicians and scientists alone. Chapters 4 and 5 will address these points in much more detail.

During the October 28, 2009 hearing, Representative Linda Sánchez (a Democrat from California) was unquestionably the most skeptical of Goodell's testimony. In her interrogation of Goodell, she expressly compares the NFL to the tobacco industry. Beginning by noting the NFL's "sort of blanket denial or minimizing of the fact that there may be this, you know, link," she moved on to identify the common rhetorical and political strategy that is the Manufacture of Doubt: "And it sort of reminds me of the tobacco companies pre-1990s when they kept saying no, there is no link between smoking and damage to your health or ill health effects."[36] Representative Sánchez then asks Goodell why it would not be better if the NFL "just embraced that there is research that suggests this and admitted to it?"[37] Goodell first professes confusion as to the question, and then asserts that "what we are doing is because we have to a large extent driven this issue by making sure that we have medical professionals studying this issue. I am not a medical professional."[38]

Further on in the exchange between Representative Sánchez and Goodell, the latter again uses a classic technique in the Manufacture of Doubt by implying that the existence of scientific debate invalidates any efforts to regulate the harm posed by occupational hazards of the industry in question:

The doctors that we have involved with this, I do not judge whether they have a particular view going in or going out. This is a collective group that are tremendous professionals, that have studied this and other issues on a scientific basis, and this is part of medical debate. And I think it is clear today there is a significant medical debate about the impact, what that impact is, and at what point.[39]

During the October 28, 2009 hearing, more than one member of the Judiciary Committee requested the testimony of Ira Casson, who had succeeded Pellman as chair of the NFL-TBIC. Casson was a lightning rod for controversy given his vocal denials of the existence of a causal link between tackle football, TBI, and severe neuropathology. Representative Conyers opened the October 28, 2009 hearing by noting that "Dr. Ira Casson, the co-chair of the NFL's Mild Traumatic Brain Injury Committee, denied the linkage on six separate occasions. When asked whether there was any linkage between playing football and CTE, Dr. Casson stated it had never been scientifically, validly documented."[40] Accordingly, a follow-up hearing was held on January 4, 2010, where Casson stated his position immediately during his prepared remarks: "My position is that there is not enough valid, reliable, or objective scientific evidence at present to determine whether or not repeat head impacts in professional football result in long-term brain damage."[41] In response to a question from Representative Sánchez, Casson demonstrates one of the paradigmatic arguments used by industrial defendants to manufacture doubt, asserting the difference between correlation and causation: "It is accepted in the sport of boxing. It's accepted in a few other circumstances. It's not necessarily generally accepted in all the football players. Now, have there been a few cases that maybe it's true? Yes. But we need more evidence. Just because there's an association does not prove causation."[42]

The tackle football industry's efforts to manufacture doubt by challenging causation did not end with these hearings. In 2018, the coach for the University of North Carolina, publicly stated, "I don't think it's been proven that the game of football causes CTE. We don't really know that." And "Are there chances for concussions? Of course. There are collisions. But the game is safer than it's ever been."[43] There are two script-making characteristics evident in this quote. The first is the causation challenge, and the second is the claim that through relevant changes in practice and in the application of novel technologies, the dangerous product can be made sufficiently safe. After the predictable outcry, the coach backed down a bit from his stance, stating subsequently, "I completely understand that there is a link between CTE and football."[44] But other commentators offered support even for his initial position: "I totally agree with him," Peter Cummings, a forensic pathologist and neuropathologist, said days after the coach's remarks. "Association is not causation. CTE has also been found in individuals not exposed to contact sports. It's not a settled matter by any means."[45]

In a 2016 article, journalists Fainaru and Fainaru-Wada interviewed neurosurgeon Uzma Samadani, who has worked as an "unaffiliated sideline consultant with the NFL." Samadani

> said she believes the league has been correct in its prior statements that no firm connection has been established between football-related head trauma and CTE—at least among youths.
>
> "We know that repetitive trauma causes CTE," Samadani said. "We've seen that in boxers. . . . I don't necessarily believe that football at the amateur level is sufficient to cause repetitive brain injury that can result in CTE."
>
> Samadani, whose recent [coauthored] book, *The Football Decision*, addresses how parents should weigh the risks of contact sports, said until researchers are able to study football players over time, including issues such [as] genetics and substance abuse, it will be impossible to assert whether head trauma is the main cause of CTE in football.[46]

Even some tackle football insiders have advised that the NFL should consider diminishing its eager use of this characteristic of the Manufacture of Doubt. Julian Bailes is a former team physician for the NFL's Pittsburgh Steelers who has been a long-term and outspoken critic of the idea that tackle football causes long-term neuropathology (and has testified as such in a variety of tort litigation). He is also the chairman of the Medical Advisory Committee for Pop Warner, the governing body for youth football in the US. But in 2016 Bailes said he thought it was dangerous for the NFL, given its influence, to continue questioning the CTE research. "We can't let these scientific discussions be hijacked by people creating doubts about causation. . . . The only known cause we have thus far is repetitive cranial impact."[47]

As an insider, Bailes's reservations about the NFL's conduct are not evidence against the applicability of this script-making characteristic—rather, they are further proof of its force and relevance. Bailes would not have made the comments he did unless he understood the NFL's long-standing behavior of attempting to deny a causal link between participation in tackle football and long-term neuropathology. The context is clear: it is dangerous for the NFL to continue to try to cast doubts about causation in particular. As an insider, Bailes well understands the significance of this particular component of the Manufacture of Doubt, as well as the extent to which the tackle football industry has used it.

Manufacture doubt by using anatomical evidence to undermine injury/illness claims

The application of this particular script-making characteristic to the tackle football industry is complex. Historically, workers and consumers who complained of illness and injury resulting from the production or consumption of the relevant product were liable to have their claims challenged by use of anatomical or morphological evidence. Recall that the railroad industry drew heavily on the absence of discernible lesions to challenge injury claims; the silica and rock–dust producing industries used X-rays for similar effect.

But as to tackle football, the "polarity" of the anatomical evidence is essentially reversed: it points strongly in favor of a causal link between workers and participants' exposure to the product. Indeed, as noted in chapter 1, contemporary debate on US tackle football and TBI exploded in 2006, when Pittsburgh-based forensic neuropathologist Bennet Omalu published a paper demonstrating CTE in the brain of Mike Webster. Since then, extensive neuroanatomical evidence, collected by a group of investigators centered at Boston University and led by scientist Ann McKee, has documented so-called tau protein pathology—considered strong evidence of CTE—in the brains of literally hundreds of former tackle football players. While most of the players who donated their brain had played in the NFL, there are also multiple findings of tau pathology in the brains of players who never played in the NFL (i.e., in the brains of former college and even high school players).[48] There is also a body of evidence documenting ominous structural and anatomical changes in the brains of youths and adolescents who play tackle football, even in the absence of a diagnosed concussion.[49] This finding is enormously important insofar as it suggests that mere participation in tackle football is associated with changes inimical to long-term neurological health, to say nothing of the additional forms of injury almost certainly caused by participation in tackle football.

In short, for a variety of reasons, anatomical evidence has generally not been especially useful for the tackle football industry's efforts to manufacture doubt. However, such evidence has still proved extremely important in the overall debate and conversation linking participation in tackle football to adverse health. Indeed, some people, such as journalists Daniel Engber and Stefan Fatsis, have argued that the overwhelming focus on neuroanatomy is problematic given the extent to which injuries and morbidities other than severe neuropathology are associated with playing tackle football.[50] But this argument would be unnecessary if the anatomical evidence of CTE were deemed unimportant or of little probative value. Anatomical evidence remains a critical tool in debates over regulated industries' public health impact; in the case of TBI and tackle football, those developing the evidence base of a causal link between exposure and harm have managed to harness such evidence. The NFL and other sophisticated actors interested in manufacturing doubt have thus been placed on the defensive as to this particular script-making characteristic rather than being able to wield it to manufacture doubt.

In particular, the NFL has followed two principal strategies for discrediting or undermining the evidence of severe neuropathology that flows from postmortem anatomical investigations of former players' brains. First, they have fallen back on the causation arguments discussed previously. While it is true that an overwhelming majority of the brains examined by McKee and her colleagues have showed clear evidence of CTE, such evidence is only correlative (i.e., the brains are associated with participation in tackle football). Critics say there is nothing about such evidence that establishes that the participation in football caused CTE. I have considered such claims in the previous section and will address them to a much greater extent in chapters 5 and 6. Relying on such arguments to delay political or legal action is a core feature of the Manufacture of Doubt.

Second, the tackle football industry, and especially the NFL, have pointed out the significant selection bias associated with the many samples investigated by McKee and her colleagues. That is, because virtually everyone who chooses to donate their brain for postmortem scientific investigation has reason to believe they are experiencing the symptoms of brain injury during life, the samples on which McKee relies are heavily skewed (i.e., it would be shocking if a large percentage of the brains did not display evidence of neurological trauma). Without having access to the full denominator of participants, it is very difficult to discern the actual prevalence of CTE and other severe neuropathologies. Here again the tackle football industry is drawing on the rhetorical and social power of anatomical evidence—the suggestion is that such power can be beguiling and dangerous insofar as it encourages people to overlook the problems with the evidence base itself.

The bias in the samples providing the anatomical evidence is undeniable. However, in an important study, Zachary O. Binney and Kathleen E. Bachynski used a number of epidemiological techniques to correct such bias and to derive a more accurate estimate of the true prevalence of CTE among NFL players (at least 10%, figuring conservatively).[51] Moreover, in a 2022 study, LeClair and colleagues adjusted for the selection bias problem in donated brains. Their work showed that estimates of CTE prevalence was actually higher after adjustment than before, meaning that the "conventional estimates were biased towards the null."[52] In other words, contrary to popular belief, the investigators found that selection bias was not artificially inflating the prevalence. They also found a dose-response relationship between the exposure (playing football) and the outcome (CTE), meaning that professional players who presumably had longer exposure periods had a higher likelihood of developing CTE.[53]

Regardless of the merits of the substantive debate, the relevant question here is the extent to which the NFL and the tackle football industry in general has used anatomical evidence to manufacture doubt. And while most of the evidence has been used by actors working to diminish such doubt, that has not prevented the tackle football industry from seizing on the power of anatomical evidence to generate what doubt can be introduced. Therefore, it is fair to say that even when faced with evidence that tilts in favor of a causal connection between exposure and harm, the tackle football industry has still found a way to use that evidence in the service of doubt.

Manufacture doubt by flooding the public arena with misleading or irrelevant data

We discuss this script-making characteristic together with the next one because both characteristics depend on sponsoring scientific research.

Manufacture doubt by hiring or partnering with officials and experts

For purposes of convenience, these two script-making characteristics have been combined. This is not because they are identical; there are many ways in which regulated industries can flood the public arena with misleading or irrelevant data. Yet virtually all such methods depend on sponsoring scientific research, which historically has tended to include partnerships with academics and public health officials that then result in ostensibly scholarly reports and publications in the peer-reviewed literature. Indeed, some regulated industries, such as the pharmaceutical industry, have perfected the use of scientific and biomedical research and publication in advancing their commercial aims. Indeed, the pharmaceutical industry's efforts have been so successful they have been described as a form of "ghost management" in which the industry's significant role in producing the relevant data is erased from public view.[54] One of the most powerful tools for skewing scientific literature is to simply refuse to publish or report so-called negative trials, or studies in which the drug product being tested does not meet the required standards for proof of efficacy.

Refusing to publish negative trials is an enormous problem that results in a powerful tool of agnotology (the construction of ignorance) termed "publication bias."[55] Consider an example where researchers conduct a total of 25 trials intended to evaluate the safety and efficacy of drug X, and 21 of them are negative with the other 4 being positive. If 20 of the negative trials are simply buried and only one of them is published, along with all 4 of the positive trials, the scientific literature will display an obvious bias towards efficacy that is totally unreflective of the actual state of the evidence. Because of the close connections between flooding the public arena with misleading data, the sponsorship of scientific and epidemiological research, and partnerships with academic scientists and public health officials, it makes sense to discuss these script-making characteristics in tandem.

The tackle football industry has without question used all of these techniques. As noted earlier, the NFL has sponsored research and investigation into the links between tackle football and injuries of all kinds (with a special focus on long-term neuropathology). The industry's efforts in these areas are significant and problematic, both from the perspective of scientific knowledge and from the perspective of social and political action.

Consider the drama that unfolded in the pages of the journal *Neurosurgery*, one of the flagship periodicals in its field. In its July 2005 issue, the journal published a paper by Bennett Omalu and colleagues presenting the results of the autopsy of the brain of former NFL player Mike Webster (who died by suicide).[56] The November 2006 issue of *Neurosurgery* featured a scathing critique of the paper; the authors of the critique argued that the paper perpetrated a "serious misconception," and they denied the finding of CTE.[57] The authors urged Omalu and colleagues to "retract their paper or sufficiently revise it and its title after detailed investigation of the case."[58] The authors of this letter, Ira R. Casson, Elliot J. Pellman, and David C. Viano, were all members of the NFL-TBIC at the time they submitted the letter. Of the six responses to the critique letter, several correspondents objected to the tone and apparent lack of "collegial respect" in the letter. Kenneth Kutner, team neuropsychologist for the New York Giants, noted that

> Casson et al.'s letter seems to have exceeded the protocol for scientifically providing an additional opinion for a published story. Specifically, they took an extreme stand in actually urging the authors to retract the article. Their stand is quite excessive, and, in my opinion, inappropriate. Articles should be considered for retraction if they contain fabricated data, contamination of data, or allegation of misconduct. It is my opinion that there is no justification for retracting this article.[59]

The NFL's own sponsored studies at this time suffered from a host of methodological problems, including missing and/or opaque data. The NFL refused to fund any studies not expressly commissioned by its sponsoring body, NFL Charities. Pressure mounted on the NFL to alter its practices, especially following the disastrous 2009 and 2010 hearings that made clear the connection to the tobacco industry forged through the Manufacture of Doubt. The NFL changed the structure of its Traumatic Brain Injury Committee and pledged both to increase the overall amount of funding it provided for research on TBI and to channel it through ostensibly neutral bodies.

The NFL committed to funding National Institutes of Health (NIH) studies on TBI, but it later pulled US$16 million in funding from the NIH over a dispute regarding whether the NFL had the right to influence "specific research funding decisions."[60] The decision sparked an immediate furor, spurring Congress to hold hearings and produce a 91-page report on the question of whether the NFL "improperly attempt[ed] to influence the grant selection process at NIH."[61] This is an accurate, somewhat brutal, demonstration of the difficulty of sticking to ethically preferable policies when they are not commercially favorable.

In 2012, the NFL donated US$30 million to the National Institute for Neurological Disorders and Stroke (NINDS) to establish the Sports Health Research Program. After two years of attempting to recruit additional funders, the director of NINDS, Walter Koroshetz, exchanged emails with Ellen Sigal, head of the nonprofit foundation Friends of Cancer Research. Their conversation was reported by a journalist.

> "Somewhat surprisingly," Koroshetz wrote to Sigal . . . , "we haven't been able to recruit other partners."
>
> He then wrote something that the rest of the world suspected but didn't know for sure at the time: "NFL not a real partner. Their agenda doesn't match ours."
>
> "Walter, this does not surprise me at all," Sigal replied. "They are real thugs who have a very low bar for anything but making money and creating violence. They were just doing this for the PR value."
>
> Koroshetz replied, "Agree. But we did get $30 million for TBI research. And we have funded very interesting projects. So NIH won this one."[62]

In the fall of 2015, the partnership completely unraveled. The NFL backed out of a specific commitment to fund a seven-year, US$16 million study of CTE because it did not agree with the NIH's award determination. The NIH had awarded the grant to a team led by Robert Stern at the Chronic Traumatic Encephalopathy Center at Boston University (the same center at which Ann McKee works; McKee and Stern were close colleagues at the time). Although the NFL had insisted that it exercised no influence over NIH award determinations, it nevertheless objected to the decision and pulled its funding. NINDS essentially shrugged its shoulders and funded the proposed research anyway. Fainaru and Fainaru-Wada reported that

> when the NFL's "unrestricted" $30 million gift was announced in 2012, the NIH said the money came "with no strings attached"; however, an NIH official clarified the gift terms two years later, telling [ESPN's] *Outside the Lines* that, in fact, the league retained veto power over projects that it funds. Koroshetz affirmed that this week. Sources told *Outside the Lines* that the league exercised that power when it learned that Stern, a professor of neurology and neurosurgery at Boston University, would be the project's lead researcher. The league, sources said, raised concerns about Stern's objectivity, despite the merit review and a separate evaluation by a dozen high-level experts assembled by the NIH.[63]

While the subject of conflicts of interest is important enough to be the focus of chapter 4, this example is important on multiple levels. The history detailed in this chapter makes plain the significance for regulated industries of partnering with academics and public health officials in the Manufacture of Doubt. Although there are many motivations for doing so, one of the most important is the need to acquire a form of social credibility. One of the inevitable costs of manufacturing doubt is the extent to which it diminishes public trust and regard for the industry in question. While the Manufacture of Doubt may be an effective regulatory and political strategy, over time public audiences tend to notice the extent to which industrial efforts in this vein corrupt analysis and policy, not to mention the often-significant ensuing public health consequences.

Thus, public opinion on the trustworthiness of regulated industries has tended to suffer over time and to the extent the industry actively attempts to construct ignorance. In her important work on the history of the partnerships between the US pharmaceutical industry and US physicians, Dominique Tobbell traces the industry's efforts to purchase social credibility through relationships with physicians as far back as the 1920s.[64] However, she documents a dramatic increase in these efforts in the post–World War II era; not coincidentally, this chronology also marks the rise of partnerships between the tobacco industry and physicians in the US and in the UK in particular.

The tackle football industry has continued to develop such partnerships in the production of reports, press statements, research, and scientific papers that "flood the public arena with misleading or irrelevant data" and thereby help to manufacture doubt. Consider, for example, the NFL's partnership with the CDC Foundation, a nonprofit organization affiliated with the CDC (Centers for Disease Control and Prevention) but legally and organizationally distinct. As Bachynski and I noted in 2018, the NFL's interests influenced the CDC's framing of the risks of sports-related brain trauma:

> In 2011 the NFL provided a grant to the CDC Foundation. The funds supported the CDC's development of Heads Up, a national educational initiative with multiple partners designed to inform healthcare professionals, educators, sports coaches, parents and youth athletes about TBIs in sports (a distinct programme from the Heads Up tackling initiative). The president and CEO of the CDC Foundation explained, "We are pleased that this public–private partnership between CDC and the NFL will expand knowledge of concussion prevention and treatment for kids and teens."[65]

The NFL exploited this connection with the CDC Foundation in its safety marketing materials:

> As a consequence of the league's involvement and financial support, the NFL's logo is emblazoned on several of the CDC's educational Heads Up fact sheets. Promoting the NFL's brand through public health agency material is a way that the league purchases credibility for its efforts. . . . The NFL has specifically pointed to its partnership with the CDC to deflect

criticism of the league's questionable research and alleged ties to the tobacco industry.[66]

At the time Bachynski and I published this paper, the CDC on its
own website hosted "materials promoting the NFL's perspective on concussions for players of all ages, notably an NFL video on safety in youth
sports featuring league Commissioner Roger Goodell."[67] These materials
were taken down within weeks of the publication of the paper, although
there is no evidence, beyond the chronology, to suggest a causal link.
The problem, however, is that the materials developed by the NFL–CDC
Foundation initiative are misleading at best. From our 2017 paper:

> [The materials] ignore public health evidence that tackling poses inherent
> risks of repeated brain trauma that cannot be prevented by player educa-
> tion, post-injury concussion management or other techniques. The fact
> sheets also endorse an approach to sports-related brain trauma that sub-
> tly deflects responsibility away from sports leagues and onto individual
> youth players and their caregivers. At issue is the way in which the NFL
> and its allies seek to frame public health messaging related to the risks of
> playing football. Regulated industries implicated in promoting dangerous
> products have often sought to delay public health action by acknowledg-
> ing the risks of their product but arguing that responsible use by end
> users and consumers can effectively mitigate these risks. In partnering
> with the NFL, the CDC is promoting materials that employ a similar strat-
> egy to the tobacco industry's efforts to shift attention away from corpo-
> rate responsibility.[68]

The NFL's efforts in this social space continue unabated. In late summer 2017, Fainaru-Wada and Fainaru reported that almost none of the
NFL's US$100 million commitment (made in 2016) to TBI research was
directed towards sponsoring research on CTE. The NFL apparently did
fund a single study on CTE, a study that

> focused on jockeys. . . . The study is led by an Australian researcher who
> once described American coverage of CTE as "carry-on and hoo-hah" and

a British doctor whose concussion presentations sometimes have included flippant jokes and video of tumbling jockeys set to slapstick music. At one presentation, the widow of a CTE victim, a former British soccer star, was so offended she stormed out of the room.[69]

The journalists note a reason for questioning the relevance of this study for American tackle football players: while jockeys may be likely to experience TBI in a fall, they generally are not subject to the persistent accumulation of insults, including subconcussive impacts, that are strongly correlated with long-term neuropathology such as CTE.[70] In any event, the NFL has made clear that it is in complete control of the US$40 million portion of the commitment it has designated for sponsoring scientific research, and given the NFL's behavior with the retracted NIH funding, there is every reason to think that the tackle football industry will continue to use the scientific publication process to manufacture doubt. Likely, no funds will be allocated to McKee, Stern, or other scientists affiliated with the Center for CTE at Boston University.

The remaining US$60 million of the "Play Smart, Play Safe" campaign is devoted to a different area of research: the engineering, production, and sale of better helmets. The focus on "superior" novel technology is itself a component of the next script-making characteristic we look at.

Manufacture doubt by claiming to design and sell a significantly "safer" version of the product

The claim that "the game is safer than it has ever been" is rampant in conversation about American tackle football. A Boolean search of North American periodicals between 2017 and 2022 for "football" and "safer" reveals over 11,000 hits, although not all of these will be relevant. For a more immediate look, simply typing the words "safer than it has ever been" in an internet search engine produces tackle football–related results in 4 out of the top 10 hits (including 2 of the top 4 hits). In October 2019, New York became one of the latest states to consider an outright ban on youth football. In opposition, the CEO of USA Football testified before the state legislature, stating that "today's game is safer than ever before. . . . [G]reater education around safety and concussions is the 'new normal.'"[71]

The appeal of the claim is obvious. It does not require denial of an established body of evidence connecting consumption of end use of the product in question to significant population health harms. Quite the contrary, it acts rhetorically to co-opt such evidence, using it as a platform on which to build a structure in relief—an edifice composed of the new, improved, safer version of the relevant product. As ever, the objective of the effort is to create, advance, or at least sustain a regulatory vacuum. If the industry can convince regulators, policymakers, and the public that a previously hazardous product has been made "sufficiently" safe, there is less reason to implement new governance strictures that could interfere with or undermine commerce. This script-making characteristic is thus important in the Manufacture of Doubt and is used often. The most successful usage has already been discussed: the tobacco industry's winning efforts to convince a skeptical public and government(s) that so-called low-tar cigarettes ushered in a new era of sufficiently safe tobacco products and consumption. Chapter 2 has also detailed the ways in which the silica and rock–dust producing industry consistently deployed this claim or close variations thereof to delay and forestall significant regulatory action for decades. Histories of the automobile industry's use of the Manufacture of Doubt reveal consistent reliance on this script-making characteristic since at least the early 1970s.[72] While the validity of the claim will be addressed in chapter 6, for now it is sufficient simply to note that the tackle football industry continues to deploy this script-making characteristic.

Helmet technology and the manufacture of doubt

The insistence that new and improved technology can save consumers from the harms caused by a hazardous industrial product is both part and parcel of this particular script-making characteristic and is of significant importance even outside of the Manufacture of Doubt. It has been termed the "technological imperative," or the notion that we can resolve any particular social problems we may have, including health problems, through application of better technology. Scholars and commentators have repeatedly documented both the manifestation of and the problems arising from the technological imperative.[73] The central issue is the effort to reduce complex social problems to technical difficulties, thereby implying they can and should be resolved simply by application of better technologies. Although better technologies can assist in a wide variety of social contexts, the idea that high-level social problems are essentially reducible to technical gaps has repeatedly proven to be a significant mistake. For example, overwhelming epidemiologic evidence shows that the prime determinants of health in human populations are the social and economic conditions in which we live, work, and play. Addressing problems in these domains requires significant changes in the way different societies organize themselves and share available goods and resources. Yet in the US, we expend overwhelming amounts of money on novel technologies that are used at the point-of-care itself, far downstream from the much larger impact that social and economic structures exert on health outcomes. Such technologies may or may not be useful in any individual case, but there is little evidence that they can affect the upstream factors that are principally responsible for driving health outcomes. Moreover, novel technologies tend to be extremely expensive, at least initially, which means that even where they may have a demonstrable impact on population health, they also tend to expand health inequalities. Because we have a basic moral obligation to act in ways that contract rather than expand existing social inequalities, this is a further reason for doubting that application of better technologies is a true health priority.

The emphasis on the role of technological interventions serves a particular risk frame. If technological interventions can substantially reduce the risk of brain injury, it follows that the game is either sufficiently safe (and has simply been played in ways that increase the risk) or can be made as such. And, if the proper application of technology can make play substantially safer, the responsibility for safety rests with the individuals who have the capacity to implement and require the use of such technology rather than with the institutional actors commodifying and selling play itself.

Chapter 6 will consider some of these points in further detail, but there is little doubt that the American tackle football industry has and continues to invest heavily in this particular component of the claim to design and sell a significantly safer version of the product in question. The tackle football industry's particular efforts here highlight the significance of (1) better technology, especially helmets; and (2) rule changes. Regarding (1), a significant amount of funding provided by the tackle football industry has gone to research on helmets.

The history regarding helmet technology is complex but significant. In both ice hockey and in American tackle football, helmets have long been touted as an essential form of protection against injuries, including concussions. For decades, the salvation of football has been attributed to the introduction and refinement of protective gear. For instance, in 1950 a columnist for the *Chicago Tribune* asserted that the football of the early twentieth century had been rendered far less dangerous "when the players were compelled to wear head-gear, braced shoes, and pads. If such protective measures had not been adopted it is questionable whether football would have survived as one of our national sports."[74] In ice hockey, by the 1960s, both Canadian and American amateur hockey associations required their youth players to wear helmets.[75]

Interdisciplinary public health scholar Kathleen Bachynski's work is the definitive scholarship on the history and ethics of helmet technology and its use in American tackle football. In a 2019 paper, she notes Phillips Andover school physician James Roswell Gallagher's emphasis in 1948 on helmets being the "least, and perhaps the most that can be done" to protect the players from head injuries.[76] The NCAA itself first required the use of helmets in 1939, but Bachynski notes that even by the 1950s, there was doubt regarding the true protective capacity of the technology.[77] Neither hockey nor football regulatory bodies imposed standards on helmet design until 1969, and the equipment in fact offered only limited protection. Two teenaged hockey players from New Brunswick suffered fatal injuries in 1968 despite having worn helmets; their deaths drew particular attention to the equipment's inadequacy. Describing these cases and noting that the helmets only protected the upper part of the skull, physician John Fekete argued in 1968 that they did "not have enough rigidity to give adequate protection against any but the slightest blow," emphasizing that "the so-called protective helmet of amateur hockey players gives only limited protection, even in minor accidents." Participants at a 1968 conference addressing sports injuries advocated the universal use of helmets while noting the inability of existing headgear to adequately prevent injuries: "Every hockey player should wear a helmet. Most, perhaps all, helmets now available, are inadequate in view of the forces involved."[78] Helmets were thus promoted as essential pieces of equipment even as their limitations were increasingly recognized.

More specifically, several key actors are worth mentioning, as their respective roles are easily scripted by the Manufacture of Doubt and are core to regulatory capture. Public health law, and tort litigation in particular, is also part of the narrative history here. It is also a key feature in the Manufacture of Doubt. Bachynski recounts the publicity surrounding Ernie Pelton, a California high school football player who in 1967 became a quadriplegic following a head injury experienced during play. His father sued the helmet manufacturer, Rawlings, arguing "that Rawlings could have made a safer helmet." Rawlings called star professional football player O. J. Simpson as a witness; Simpson testified that he "believe[d] in this helmet."[79]

[The] Sacramento jury . . . sent a note to the judge asking for the star's autograph. After an 89-day hearing, the jury cleared the manufacturer of any responsibility for Ernie's injury. The president of Rawlings not only celebrated the outcome for his company, but also suggested the future of the sport had turned on the case. "Football was on trial at Sacramento." Meanwhile, Ernie would never walk again.[80]

Beginning in the 1960s, a number of entities jockeyed for position as the leading authority on helmet standards. The clear winner emerged in the 1970s: the National Operating Committee on Standards for Athletic Equipment (NOCSAE). Bachynski explains the reasons why. First, NOCSAE was from inception a creature of leading sports organizations, including the NCAA and the National Federation of State High School Associations (NFHS). "These organizations' involvement in NOCSAE was intended to ensure that they could retain control over sports standards, rules, and regulations."[81] Second, none of these member sports organizations paid any dues; all the funding for NOCSAE was supplied by the Sporting Goods Manufacturers Association—the trade group for helmet manufacturers. To summarize, then, part of the reason NOCSAE emerged victorious as the standard setter for tackle football helmets is because it (1) included key players in the tackle football industry, and (2) was funded by the helmet manufacturers themselves (through their trade association). Indeed, Bachynski goes on to note that an older and competing group, ASTM, "emphasized expertise in standards writing and explicitly sought to limit the influence of vested interests in sporting goods manufacturing. . . . Another ASTM rule required that the number of producers could not exceed non-producers of sports equipment on the committee."[82] These rules, presumably enacted to combat the adverse effects of COIs and motivated bias so deeply interwoven in the Manufacture of Doubt, were precisely those that helped ensure NOCSAE's victory in standards setting. Adherence to the Manufacture of Doubt thus brings significant rewards not simply to members of the regulated industry itself, but to ancillary or connected actors that enjoy sufficient overlap with the interests of the regulated industry. And the emphasis on the certification of safety standards by a "separate" organization wholly funded by regulated industry is also a script-making characteristic of the Manufacture of Doubt. In particular, the tobacco, food, pharmaceutical, and alcoholic beverage industries have made use of this technique.

Bachynski points out that the momentum towards the establishment of helmet safety standards was fueled in large part by the fear of liability from litigation:

> In 1970, *NCAA News* described the formation of NOCSAE as part of an article announcing the jury decision—a victory, from the NCAA's perspective—to clear Rawlings of any legal responsibility for a catastrophic football injury. It was the case of Ernie Pelton, the high school player who had been left quadriplegic "from a violent twisting of the head" after being tackled. Manufacturers and sports administrators emphasized the importance of legally protecting themselves in such cases, while contending that helmets were not at fault for injuries.[83]

Furthermore, "manufacturers were not motivated to develop helmet standards by the U.S. government threatening to shut down football. Rather, standards were largely prompted by a shifting legal landscape that increased manufacturers' risk of liability. Federal agencies were not threatening the existence of football, but legal trends were threatening the industry's profits."[84] Bachynski's analysis here is important on at least two grounds. First, it justifies the claim that American tackle football is a regulated industry. This may seem counterintuitive, since Bachynski is here arguing that the development and adoption of helmet standards was not precipitated by the threat of formal regulatory action. But litigation in context of occupational and industrial harm is a form of public health law. As argued above, it makes little sense to assert that the tackle football industry's success in avoiding regulation means that it is not a regulated industry. Instead, what it demonstrates is the success of the industry in creating an almost total regulatory vacuum. The existence of that vacuum produces a lack of any form of governance to curb or somehow leaven the harms flowing from the hazardous product. This vacuum prompts concerned actors, including those most at risk or actually harmed by exposure to the product, to seek other means of governance. Without an effective public law response, members of the public seeking shelter from the harms of the product may have no other option but to turn to private law—the tort liability system. (The use of litigation as a tool for public health law will be discussed in detail in chapter 6.)

Second, the ways that regulated industries manage and respond to the risks of tort liability are a consistent feature of the Manufacture of Doubt. In context of the tackle football industry, it is therefore unsurprising that this particular script-making characteristic—"technology will save us"—developed and took a specific form and pathway almost entirely in response to the many attempts to hold the industry responsible for the harms caused by the product it marketed and sold.

Sander Reynolds, vice president for product development at Xenith, a company that manufactures football helmets, admitted to *New York Times* reporter Alan Schwarz that NOCSAE ultimately "exists for two reasons—to avoid skull fractures, and to avoid liability."[85] Nonetheless, helmets continue to be portrayed and pursued as a key means of reducing TBI. NOCSAE's methods for evaluating the sufficiency of football helmets were flawed from the start. They based their entire certification system on car crash safety research that assessed only linear impacts. This is problematic because of the evidence, already emerging in the early 1970s, that "rotational motion appeared to be more critical than linear motion to the production of human brain injury."[86] In addition, Bachynski notes that NOCSAE certified refurbished helmets on the basis of a sample size of one helmet.

While acknowledging that the NOCSAE helmet standard is not a TBI standard, NOCSAE nevertheless asserts on its website that "a helmet certified to a NOCSAE standard provides a substantial level for serious head injuries, including concussions."[87] Furthermore, despite a lack of evidence, helmet manufacturers have promoted their products' ability to prevent TBI. The most recent example was Vicis, Inc., which declared bankruptcy in 2019 and was subsequently acquired by a company named Certor Sports. The company's first major product was the Zero1, a football helmet priced at US$950–US$1,700. Prior to its bankruptcy, Vicis showed care with language on its website:

> The ZERO1 has been extensively tested by the leading biomechanics labs in North America and offers better overall performance than any football helmet ever tested under today's leading protocols, which integrate both linear and rotational forces to determine helmet effectiveness.
>
> There is no scientific consensus around impact thresholds and concussion. The level of impact necessary to sustain a concussion can vary by individual, and many non-impact factors may play a role. While substantial research supports the role of impact force reduction in mitigating concussion risk and severity, neither the ZERO1 nor any other helmet can claim to reduce or eliminate concussions.[88]

Note that this statement includes: a description of their testing, which includes measures of linear and rotational forces; the admission that no helmet can claim even to reduce concussions; and language regarding the significant variability in the incidence and severity of TBI resulting from collision sports. Nevertheless, the marketing for the product emphasized the helmet's ability to "reduce head impact severity." Moreover, a Vicis infographic on their website included the emblazons of both the NFL and the NFLPA—the labor union representing the players.[89]

There is much more to be said about regulated industries' use of technology to create doubt as to the need for tighter governance of a hazardous project. But for a full and especially rich account of the social impact of helmet technology in context of tackle football, readers should closely examine Bachynski's standard-setting text.

Rule changes and the manufacture of doubt

The role that rule changes play is complex and significant. Because the tackle football industry's product is literally a game, the extent to which this particular technique is applicable to other regulated industries is unclear. There is therefore a sense in which the tackle football industry has helped to pioneer this element of the Manufacture of

Doubt. The emphasis on rule changes can be grouped with the campaign for better helmet technology by understanding how the tackle football industry is trying to frame the risk its participants face. This risk framing is important to the Manufacture of Doubt and is a way that regulated industries have fought to create or sustain a regulatory vacuum, as well as influence opinion on the relative safety and use of its products. Bachynski and I note in a 2014 paper that "the framing of risk is not a neutral, apolitical enterprise."[90] Specifically as to tackle football in the US and ice hockey in Canada,

> powerful institutional and political actors have advanced a particular framework for interpreting the risk of mTBI [mild TBI]. This framework emphasizes that play is sufficiently safe, and that the risks of the game can be reduced to acceptable levels via laws, technological interventions, and rule changes. The risk frame also implies that the risks of brain injury that seem to be correlated with play are largely the responsibility of the people most directly connected to the individual player's participation (i.e., the trainers, coaches, and of course the players themselves).[91]

Although much of the epidemiologic literature regarding football-related TBI discusses, in passing, the notion of rule changes, there is very little high-quality evidence via prospective studies establishing robust correlations between rule changes and significantly reduced risk. Against that paucity of evidence, we can read institutional actors' emphasis on rule changes as a pathway to player safety and TBI risk reduction as a key plank in those actors' preferred risk frame. The idea that American tackle football can be made safe, and that the risks faced by some of the most vulnerable groups in American society can be substantially diminished, is critical to shaping public discussion on the urgent question of whether the risks involved are acceptable in exchange for the expected benefits of football play. An alternative and arguably more plausible risk frame suggests that significant risk inheres in play and in many cases cannot be substantially reduced without entirely transforming the game. This latter frame might produce a different decision calculus for families deciding whether to permit their children to play American tackle football. That is, entirely eliminating contact from the game would be likely to substantially reduce the risk. But within the context of American football as a full-contact game, limited evidence links rule changes to anything other than marginal reductions in risk. This underscores the importance of a frame that casts the fundamental question as whether the levels of risk that currently attend play are acceptable, and for whom. These difficult questions are covered in detail in chapters 4 and 5.

✕✕✕

The analysis in this chapter shows one main idea: the American tackle football industry has actively engaged in, and in many cases developed and refined, each of the eight most significant script-making characteristics that create a certain family resemblance. And the "family" in question here is the Manufacture of Doubt. Put plainly, American tackle football is a regulated industry that has consistently manufactured doubt regarding the causal connection between the use of its product (by workers and nonemployee participants) and health harms. The industry continues to do so to the present.

Chapters 1–3 form the backbone of the argument in this book. Taken together, they establish that American tackle football constitutes a regulated industry, and like many other highly profitable, regulated US industries, deploy the Manufacture of Doubt to create a regulatory vacuum. This vacuum enables the continued marketing and sale of its extremely lucrative product, but also exposes workers and nonemployee participants, including youths and adolescents, to epidemiologically significant risks of injury and morbidity.

Chapter 4 picks up the analysis at this point, focusing on a particular element of the Manufacture of Doubt: conflicts of interest. Conflicts of interest (COIs) are so rampant and so significant in effectuating the goals of the Manufacture of Doubt, they are conceptually more important than virtually any single script-making characteristic. Indeed, COIs knit together multiple script-making characteristics. Flooding the public with misleading or irrelevant data, hiring or partnering with public health officials, scientists, and physicians (including the revolving door problem discussed in chapter 4), and disputing causation all depend in important ways on the relationships that regulated industries are able to cultivate with key actors in academia and in the public sector. Moreover, this chapter has also emphasized that disputing causation is a script-making characteristic of unusual importance. Thus, where COIs are core to successful efforts to generate doubt on causation, this provides an additional reason for giving COIs the focus of a separate chapter.

4

Conflicts of Interest and the Tackle Football Industry

Conflicts of interest (COIs) are a species of what is more precisely known as "motivated bias." All humans exhibit forms of bias, which is roughly defined as an "inclination of temperament or outlook." Biases can be reasonable or unreasonable, and they exist in all humans partly because of our basic cognitive makeups and partly because we are social creatures who form relationships with each other. The latter category is especially interesting because there is a wealth of evidence demonstrating how our relationships can "motivate" us to be biased in powerful ways. These motivated biases are obviously not all problematic; few would suggest the strong emotions that motivate parents to be biased in favor of their children are inherently concerning. Yet, few would also deny that in some social contexts, those powerful motivations to exhibit bias would be problematic, as in the case where a parent must judge the winner of a music competition that includes their child.

Virtually all of us form relationships. These relationships help give our lives meaning. As a result, COIs and motivated bias are common. We cannot avoid all COIs without avoiding social life altogether. However, we do have agency to avoid or eliminate many of these sources of motivated bias, and part of the ethical issue is discerning when and why we are obligated to eliminate certain relationships that give rise to motivated bias. Thus, governors and presidents are typically required to divest their interests and relationships with private entities who stand to benefit from the power such figures wield once in office. It would be highly inappropriate for a governor to continue to serve as the CEO of an alcoholic beverage company while formally occupying public office.

COIs and motivated bias raise important ethical questions concerning which relationships we should cultivate in different social contexts. Moreover, to the extent that some people are in a social position that enables them to make decisions that have powerful consequences for people's health, those COIs can become critical issues of public health ethics. Unfortunately, just as COIs and motivated bias are common in our society, they are similarly common in the health professions. They also have an extensive history and role in the Manufacture of Doubt.

This chapter begins by exploring some of this history to frame why regulated industries have consistently utilized COIs in service of agnotology (the construction of ignorance) and the Manufacture of Doubt. It then explains how the American tackle football industry has applied these same techniques and has been riddled with extensive COIs that have motivated all sorts of health professionals to behave in biased ways that have profoundly undermined the health and well-being of players. The final portion of the chapter considers the ongoing ethical and legal implications of the COIs that abound at all levels of play and weighs legal and policy remedies for addressing COIs and motivated bias in American tackle football.

The Historical Use of Conflicts of Interest in Manufacturing Doubt

This book has repeatedly noted that COIs are an integral part of the historical Manufacture of Doubt. Why?

Chapter 2 explores several reasons for the proliferation of these conflicts. First is a structural feature of the regulatory state itself. Recall that statutes typically contain almost none of the specific details needed to render laws workable on a day-to-day basis. While the Americans with Disabilities Act may define broadly what a "reasonable accommodation is" under the law, it tells employers little about whether a specific request for a specific employee in a specific labor context is legally required. By design, legislatures delegate authority to the executive branch of government to work out these details and prescribe all the rules needed for private actors to understand how to meet the obligations imposed by a particular piece of legislation. This delegation is so common to statutes that provisions that accomplish this are referred to as "implementing" or "delegating" provisions.

Within the executive branch of government, agencies are typically the entities responsible for implementing legislation. Unlike legislators, who are only rarely subject-matter experts in the specific content of a law, the people who work at agencies are frequently trained experts on the industries they regulate. Indeed, regulators must maintain such expertise, as it would be impossible to craft meaningful rules absent a keen understanding of the industries and commerce to be regulated. Moreover, the nature of regulatory work means that regulators often have relatively frequent contact with the industries they are charged with regulating. For example, the process of developing rules and regulations that govern industrial behavior is often impossible to complete without some consultation with the industry itself. Thus, industries participate vigorously in the "notice and comment" period that agencies are required to maintain before codifying rules. Regulatory hearings and administrative appeals also involve engagement with industrial actors. Because motivated bias and COIs are primarily a function of our relationships, it is unsurprising that the relatively close relationships many regulators have with the industries being regulated lead to significant problems with motivated bias and COIs.

Chapter 2 notes that a second reason for the proliferation of COIs in the Manufacture of Doubt is because professional experts are often crucial in advancing industrial aims and objectives. Sometimes, these objectives are concrete and practical, as with the railroad and mining industry's efforts to kneecap injury or illness claims brought by workers. Physicians in particular were essential to accomplishing these goals, which is why they were directly hired by the industries under at least partial pretense of providing care for the workers. (COIs and motivated bias are often complex, precisely because people can simultaneously pursue multiple goals that exist in tension. Industry physicians might well have wanted to heal and care for injured or sick workers, at the same time they had motivations to bias their opinions and protocols in favor of their employers. This is characteristic of COIs in general.)

But in terms of larger political and social debates over industrial harm, regulated industries sought relationships with health professionals, scientists, and former regulators for an additional reason: to purchase credibility. Participating in the Manufacture of Doubt is not without its drawbacks. Such participation essentially requires working within the spheres of public reason and debate. And over time, the public typically begins to notice what the regulated industry is doing. Seeing industrial efforts to sow doubt and skepticism regarding the health harms of their products has the distinct tendency to erode public trust. This erosion of public trust is quite problematic to regulated industries' political and economic aims. For example, experts in business valuation routinely point out that often the most valuable component of a company is not how many units it sells, its annual revenues, or its market penetration. Rather, what is often most valuable is goodwill—how the company is perceived by its customers. Consumers who adore particular brands or companies will tend over time to affirm that feeling; these affirmations, if repeated in hundreds, thousands, or millions of customers, do more to advance a company's bottom line than any snapshots or metrics of financial health ever could. Apple is such a valuable company for precisely this reason: many of its customers absolutely love Apple products and are consistently willing to pay more for its products, partly as a function of that goodwill.

Conversely, lack of goodwill and lack of trust are problems for any industrial enterprise, but is especially problematic for companies and industries that are attempting to manufacture doubt. The task of constructing ignorance in public and political contexts is made infinitely more difficult if people simply do not trust the statements, testimony, and perspectives flowing from the industry.

Since credibility and goodwill is something that regulated industries find very difficult to manufacture at the same time they are manufacturing doubt, industries are forced to acquire credibility by other means: they purchase it from an external source. Like any intelligent buyer, regulated industries are interested in high-quality goods and services. They tend to know their market, so to speak, and they have the savvy and capital to acquire what they seek. Historically, physicians and scientists in particular enjoy such levels of public goodwill, trust, and credibility that industries like tobacco, lead, and pharmaceuticals can only dream of. Therefore, regulated industries have a long history of retaining the services of physicians and scientists as a means of acquiring credibility and trust. For example, historian Dominique Tobbell points out that close relationships between the pharmaceutical industry and physicians and scientists goes back in the US at least as far as the 1920s.[1] These relationships accelerated in the following decades, such that companies like "Eli Lilly and Merck had, by the early 1940s, developed elaborate knowledge networks with the medical community. These networks were fostered through the awarding of fellowships and grants to researchers and academic departments as well as through donations of research material to clinical researchers."[2] The pharmaceutical industry also established a robust set of consultancy agreements with academic physicians and scientists, "providing firms with advice on specific developments in their industrial laboratories and on corporate research strategy."[3]

Tobbell documents how these relationships deepened dramatically in the post–World War II era. In 1948, the president of Harvard University, Edward Reynolds, "proposed, essentially, a recruitment pipeline that would run between Harvard and Merck."[4] Moreover, in the mid-twentieth century, organized medicine and the pharmaceutical industry in the US shared a common hobgoblin: the specter of increased government oversight. The pharmaceutical industry avidly pursued the familiar

objectives of the Manufacture of Doubt—staving off laws and regulations and sustaining a regulatory vacuum. In organized medicine, they
found an eager ally in that fight, as the history of American medicine's
staunch resistance to laws and regulations governing the structure, financing, and delivery of health care is extremely well-documented.[5]

As chapter 2 documents, by 1962, sufficient concern over the safety
and efficacy of pharmaceuticals (including the thalidomide scandal) led
Congress to pass new legislation that dramatically impacted the pharmaceutical industry. Most notably, pharmaceutical companies now had
to seek FDA approval before they could proceed from preclinical (often
animal) studies to conducting studies with human participants. In addition, pharmaceutical companies were now required to demonstrate the
safety and efficacy of their new products, whereas in the past they had
only been required to prove safety. The industry dealt with these developments and restrictions in many of the same ways previous industries
had engaged increased federal oversight over their commercial practices:
they set up high-level commissions charged with "advising" the government and regulatory bodies charged with the oversight responsibility.
The Pharmaceutical Manufacturers Association (PMA), the trade group
for the industry, created the first of these in the summer of 1962, named
the Commission on Drug Safety.[6] Just as the Air Hygiene Control Board
set up by the foundry industry during the 1930s, industry representatives occupied a prominent place, taking up half of the membership, with
the other half being academic physicians. However, Tobbell explains, "the
Commission on Drug Safety recognized that as an industry-funded entity, it could not function effectively as a permanent advisory body;
there was a risk that its motives and the objectivity of its advice would
be questioned."[7]

Accordingly, the PMA contacted the National Research Council (of
the National Academy of Sciences) and proposed setting up, through the
Academy, a "supreme court" of pharmaceutical experts; this became
known as the Drug Research Board (DRB).[8] Tobbell points out that the
membership of this board "consisted of high-ranking industry and aca-

demic medical scientists; many of the latter also had affiliations with industry" and that

> the DRB operated for twelve years (from 1964 through 1975), during which time it was at the center of industry and academic medicine's efforts to reshape the regulatory environment to better suit their interests after the 1962 Drug Amendments. In particular, as pharmaceutical reformers in Congress pushed to further increase the government's authority over pharmaceutical practice, the DRB's work proved critical in undermining these efforts.[9]

Note that the pharmaceutical industry is both closely tracking the Manufacture of Doubt as well as refining and even pioneering new strategies for the script. While partnership with physicians and scientists predates the pharmaceutical industry, they made particularly good use of this strategy in staving off government oversight and sustaining the largest regulatory vacuum possible. Tobbell describes this relationship: "Because the government regarded academic physicians and researchers as credible experts—and interpreted academics' relations with drug firms as providing researchers with critical knowledge and insights into drug development—it [the government] routinely sought their help with the writing of pharmaceutical regulations and policy."[10] Indeed, the pharmaceutical industry enjoyed so much success in partnering with academic physicians and scientists, they managed to teach other industries the use of this particular technique in the Manufacture of Doubt. Tobbell explains that their "strategies served as a model for other industries eager to secure the guidance, expertise, and credibility of academic researchers as they fought against public criticism and expanding government regulation. The tobacco industry . . . looked to emulate the drug industry's strategy of aligning with academic researchers able to undermine the scientific legitimacy of proposed regulatory reforms."[11]

Purchasing the credibility of academic physicians and scientists therefore became an integral component of the Manufacture of Doubt in the middle decades of the twentieth century. This technique, by definition, requires close relationships between industry and physicians and scientists. Yet such relationships introduce enormous problems of COIs and motivated bias. These problems, and the devastating consequences for public health, is the subject of the following section.

Motivated Bias and Its Consequences for Public Health

Motivated bias is not an individual failing. Although we are all accountable for our actions, because we virtually all form human relationships, we are also all subject to motivated bias. Unfortunately, motivated bias can have powerful impacts on our behavior, regardless of what we intend. How?

The best model for understanding the ways in which our relationships motivate us to bias comes from political scientist Andrew Stark.[12] He suggests a three-phase model that emphasizes the ways that motivated bias and COIs unfold as part of a cognitive process. The first phase consists of "antecedent acts," which are basically any acts that solidify a relationship between the parties in question. A physician agreeing to consult or testify for a company or an industry is one example, but so are other social engagements such as having lunch with industry representatives (food and drink is a powerful glue for social relations!). Any act that brings parties into a relationship can qualify as an antecedent act under Stark's model.

The second phase is "states of mind." When the antecedent acts that bring the parties into relations are positive and enjoyable, the parties tend over time to form favorable dispositions towards each other. In and of itself, these tendencies are critical to forming social relationships of mutual support and social cohesion. We pursue relationships with each other precisely because they help give our lives meaning, and so logically, we tend to favor the people and communities that join us to form positive, nourishing relationships.

These positive states of mind lead to the third phase, which is "behavior of partiality." This is the biased or partial behavior most of us are familiar with when we think about COIs. It is the most obvious behavior of partiality that tends to make front page news, such as when a physician offering advice is revealed to have accepted large sums of money from a private company that is invested in the content of the advice. Most people tend to focus on the behavior of partiality (the last stage) because it can often be scandalous, as in the evidence from the class action litigation against opioid manufacturers revealing that physicians attended exotic dancing establishments paid for by the drug company.[13] But Stark's model reminds us that motivated bias unfolds through a sequence, with behavior of partiality only following antecedent acts that create favorable states of mind. These states of mind are the conditions that can, over time and as the relationships endures and deepens, lead to behavior of partiality.

There are a number of advantages that flow from thinking about motivated bias and COIs in terms of Stark's model.

> First, it draws from and is firmly rooted in the extensive empirical evidence regarding motivated bias. Second, it understands motivated bias as a process. Understanding COIs as a process also has a number of advantages. Like most processes, given results are not guaranteed just because prior steps occur. That is, even where antecedent acts give rise to favorable states of mind, it does not follow that behavior of partiality will occur in any given case. COIs must be understood and analyzed iteratively.

Over the long run of cases, antecedent acts that give rise to favorable states of mind are overwhelmingly likely to result in at least some behavior of partiality. In addition, understanding COIs as a process illuminates the incoherence of referring to "actual" versus "potential" COIs. COIs either exist or they do not. They exist wherever antecedent acts occur. These antecedent acts tend to give rise to favorable states of mind that in turn tend to give rise to behavior of partiality over the long run of cases. That such behavior does not occur in any given case is a feature of virtually any evidence-based framework for conceptualizing motivated bias. The occurrence of behavior of partiality does not somehow transmogrify a "potential" COI to an "actual" one. Hence, a dichotomy between "actual" and "potential" COIs makes no sense and is unmoored from the cognitive science underlying frameworks of the motivated bias.

Before applying Stark's model to the American tackle football industry, the obvious question is: Why does this matter? The answer is: "COIs and motivated bias are direct population health hazards."[14] COIs, especially when they involve regulated industries that sell dangerous products, harm people. In scientific terms, they are epidemiologic exposures, akin to any other exposure we deem adverse to health and well-being (i.e., lead, toxic solvents and chemicals, pathogens like viruses and bacteria, etc.). This is not the customary way we tend to think of COIs. Nevertheless, from a public health standpoint, the relevant question is: Do we have proof of causation linking COIs and adverse health that is generated by studies consistent with generally accepted methods in epidemiologic science? And what does such proof consist of? In the context of the pharmaceutical industry, for example, the evidence is overwhelming that deep professional–industry relationships result in significant behavioral changes (including increases in prescribing specific drugs).[15]

These increased prescriptions are strongly linked with adverse health; one prominent example is the first wave of the opioid poisoning crisis between 2009–2012.[16] Thus, the chain of inference goes from professional–industry relationships, to increased prescriptions, to clinically meaningful negative outcomes (i.e., harm) in a relatively large population. The evidence linking COIs to changes in health professional behavior is solid. The evidence linking these changes to harm in a given population is also solid. This is more than sufficient, under ordinary epidemiologic standards, to license a causal inference.[17]

While a particular COI may not cause behavior of partiality in any individual case, in the long run of cases, deep relationships between health professionals and regulated industries have caused significant harm to many vulnerable populations. Physicians and epidemiologists in particular were instrumental in the tobacco industry's efforts to manufacture doubt. As David Michaels notes, the tobacco industry's incredible success in sowing doubt forestalled regulatory action for decades, re-sulting in sickness and death for millions of people—a great proportion of which could have been prevented had governance begun in earnest in the 1950s or 1960s.[18] This is harm, and historians of the tobacco indus-try highlight the importance of health professional and scientist part-nership with the industry in causing such harm.[19]

One additional emerging framework that highlights the connections between COIs and health outcomes is known as the "commercial de-terminants of health" (CDoH) concept. According to Ilona Kickbusch and colleagues, CDoH are "strategies and approaches used by the pri-vate sector to promote products and choices that are detrimental to health."[20] The CDoH framework acknowledges the historically power-ful effects that commercial actors have on public health and, consistent with the epidemiologic analysis noted above, elevates commercial ac-tors to the level of determinants of population health. Melissa Mialon proposes an integrated model of the pathways between commercial activity and adverse population health centering on three components: (1) unhealthy commodities; (2) business, market, and political practices; and (3) global drivers (e.g., market-driven economies, trade agreements, etc.).[21] The CDoH framework has been applied to a number of regulated industries, including but not limited to the tobacco industry, the phar-maceutical industry, and global food conglomerates such as the sugar-sweetened beverage industry[22] and the commercial milk industry.[23]

Ultimately, COIs matter because they are important determinants of health. They can cause serious harm. We ought to take them seriously in any public health context, and this includes American tackle football.

Conflicts of Interest and the American Tackle Football Industry

As to American tackle football, we can begin by noting a deeply problematic structure: the health professionals charged with protecting the well-being of players are typically contracted and paid directly by the team or the league itself. This model of care begins at the top, with the

NFL. In the NFL, team physicians and trainers are contracted by and paid directly by the teams themselves. While most of them are not employees of the NFL teams for whose players they care, the physicians still contract with and are compensated directly by the teams themselves. Indeed, one team of scholars noted in 2016 that under the then-current NFL's Medical Sponsorship Policy, physicians were expressly permitted to pay NFL teams directly for the right to provide health care services for the team's players.[24]

The NFL might be the only multibillion-dollar corporation in the US that still sponsors a model of health care pioneered by the railroad industry. The COIs and motivated bias are obvious, but Stark's model is still worth applying. The formal existence of a contractor relationship in which physicians, trainers, and health professionals are paid directly by the teams easily satisfies the first stage (antecedent acts). These antecedent acts solidify a relationship with the professional team itself, which leads to the second stage, states of mind favorable to the interests of the team. Over time, these favorable dispositions tend to lead to the third stage, behavior of partiality in favor of the team interests rather than in service of the individual patient.

The evidence for the relevance of the model, and indeed the behavior of partiality from NFL-affiliated health professionals, is overwhelming. Fainaru and Fainaru-Wada's book *League of Denial* explicitly documents some of these findings,[25] as does the testimony and documents filed in support of the NFL concussion litigation. The root of the concerns over COIs and motivated bias are that team health professionals, like the railway surgeons before them, are directly paid by the teams that have a vested interest in returning sick or injured workers to play as soon as possible. The reports of this behavior are legion. For decades, NFL players have consistently described the enormous pressure they face from coaches and team officials to return to practice or games regardless of the extent of their injury. During the October 28, 2009 congressional hearing on football head injuries, Gay Culverhouse, the daughter of the original owner of the Tampa Bay Buccaneers, and a doctorally trained expert in special education, describes the conflict in no uncertain terms:

> One of the things you, as a Committee, need to understand very clearly is the fact that the team doctor is hired by the coach and paid by the front office. This team doctor is not a medical advocate for the players. This team doctor's role is to get that player back on the field, even if that means injecting the player on the field. I have seen a wall of players surround a player, a particular player, and seen his knees injected, seen his hip injected between plays and him back on the field. This is inexcusable. And I want you to understand the role that the medical community has in facilitating these concussions.[26]

During a game on December 8, 2011, a player named James Harrison tackled another player named Colt McCoy. McCoy lay on the field after the play. Replays plainly showed that the brunt of the impact had been taken on or near McCoy's head. Team trainers helped McCoy to the sideline. Exactly two plays later, McCoy returned to the field and played for the rest of the game. McCoy told reporters after the game that he neither remembered the tackle nor much of the game; "reporters were asked to turn off the lights on their cameras" while asking him questions. Journalist Chris Mortensen subsequently reported that no one on the team's training or medical staff administered the standard concussion test until the following morning, at which time it revealed "abnormal results." A representative of the NFL Players' Association reportedly told Mortensen that the event amounted to a "total system failure." Twelve days later, the NFL reversed its long-standing policy and initiated a rule requiring that trainers not affiliated with either team be seated in the press box or the coaches' box "to assist in spotting and checking for concussions." However, the policy "[stopped] short of putting independent neurologists on the sidelines to perform concussion checks."[27]

It is critical to note that the problems here have nothing to do with a particular health professional's individual virtue or goodness. Indeed, the evidence is overwhelming that motivated bias and COIs shape professional behavior regardless of physicians' commitments to behave in the best interests of their patients. As I've argued elsewhere, "the influences on behavior are extremely subtle, often working on the subconscious level to create states of mind that align with or oppose certain interests connected to the practice under consideration."[28] We do not need to assert any widespread moral failing among company physicians—that they are somehow inherently morally worse than the rest of us. Rather, the argument states that tremendously powerful social and economic forces create states of mind that lead to behavior of partiality in the aggregate. History unquestionably shows that professional participation in payment models directly sponsored by the company itself produces such behavior of partiality.

The argument from history belies the oft-cited claim that professional commitments to behave in the best interests of the patient are sufficient to preclude the effects of motivated bias on our behavior. This assertion is demonstrably false. Such commitments are necessary but totally insufficient to prevent behavior of partiality flowing from deep relationships between health professionals, scientists, and regulated industries. "The club doctor cannot always hold the player's interests as paramount and at the same time abide by his or her obligations to the club."[29]

American tackle football is violent. Serious injuries are the norm. The violence and harm its participants endure makes the health care services provided to professional players all the more significant. And the NFL, by the very structure through which health care is organized, financed, and delivered, places its workers at grave risk of motivated bias, thereby intensifying the health harms which they face. This is ethically inappropriate and should be amended. There is little serious disagreement with this notion. In 2016, a team of researchers at Harvard University funded by the NFL Players Association (NFLPA) issued a 500-page report containing 76 recommendations aimed at improving players' health. Among the most prominent of these recommendations was for the NFL to end its practice of health professionals being directly compensated by individual teams.

> The current arrangement in which club (i.e., "team") medical staff, including doctors, athletic trainers, and others, have responsibilities both to players and to the club presents an inherent conflict of interest. To address this problem and help ensure that players receive medical care that is as free from conflict as possible, division of responsibilities between two distinct groups of medical professionals is needed. Player care and treatment should be provided by one set of medical professionals (called the "Players' Medical Staff"), appointed by a joint committee with representation from both the NFL and NFLPA, and evaluation of players for business purposes should be done by separate medical personnel (the "Club Evaluation Doctor").[30]

The rationale for this recommendation is that the "division of responsibilities" will diminish the motivations a health professional might have to behave partially in favor of an individual team's interests to the possible detriment of a player's health.

The NFL roundly rejected the recommendations.

The model of COI sketched here points to only one real remedy for addressing ethical problems of COIs and motivated bias: sequestration.[31] Sequestration is generally defined as "setting apart" or "segregating." This idea matters because COIs are rampant. We all form relationships, and these relationships then motivate us to act in biased ways. How can we address these biases?

Sequestration as Remedy for Conflicts of Interest

Many people tend to think that one of the best ways to remedy the ethical problems posed by COIs is to disclose the existence of these relationships. The general theory animating this approach is known as the "sunshine theory"—that shining a light on the relationships is sufficient to remedy the ethical problems posed by COIs. Often drawing on metaphors of "sunlight" and "disinfectants," the idea is that by rendering all relationships with commercial industries visible to key stake-holders, those stakeholders can thereby 'discount' the epistemic value of the claim, evidence, diagnosis or recommendation offered by the con-flicted party. Under this theory, the problem is not that the relevant relationships exist, but is rather that if it is not disclosed, stakeholders may be unable to judge the extent to which the opinion of the conflicted party is driven by a desire to serve the interests of a party other than the key stakeholder.

Unfortunately, this theory is supported by almost no evidence in either experimental or natural conditions. To see why, consider Stark's three-stage model of COIs and motivated bias. Antecedent acts form re-lationships that lead to favorable states of mind. These favorable states of mind tend to promote behavior of partiality. The crucial question is: At what stage in this process does disclosure act to intervene? Presum-ably, if Stark's taxonomy accurately reflects the process through which COIs influence behavior, any intervention we might design ought to interfere with the process. Moreover, as a measure of the intervention's efficacy, such interference ought to occur prior to the occurrence of any behavior of partiality. Remedies that take effect only after such behav-ior has occurred are obviously suboptimal, as by that time the bad acts we presumably seek to prevent have already occurred.

The central deficiency of disclosure as a remedy is that it simply does not interfere with the three-stage process. Disclosing the existence of re-lationships between health professionals and employers does not stymie or eliminate those relationships. Where the antecedent acts exist and re-lationships form, disclosure does nothing to prevent the favorable states of mind that such relationships promote. And, where favorable states of mind are present, disclosing the existence of relationships also does nothing to prevent behavior of partiality in the long run.

Stark's theory helps explain why disclosure has repeatedly proven ineffective in preventing the ethical problems and behavior of partiality that flows from COIs. Worse yet, there is evidence that using disclosure as a remedy for such problems can actually have perverse effects and intensify behavior of partiality. There are many possible reasons for such countereffects. Patients are often reluctant to show mistrust towards health professionals and especially physicians. Thus a physician who discloses a financial relationship with a team may have players *more* likely to rely on the physician's perspective. Moreover, often people who disclose relationships at the core of COIs feel a kind of moral complacency precisely because they feel they have satisfied their moral obligations by disclosing the relevant relationships. Accordingly, providers who disclose the existence of relationships with commercial industries may feel a kind of moral license to enmesh themselves deeper in relationship with those industries, making behavior of partiality even more likely in the long run. The situation with the NFL shows this perfectly. The existence of deep relationships between teams and the health professionals who they compensate is perfectly open and transparent and has been so for decades. Nothing about this "sunshine" has obviated the extensive problems and motivated bias that the existence of these relationships alone would predict.

If the "sunshine" theory is flawed and disclosure simply does not work in preventing behavior of partiality, what does? There is only one approach that has shown any effectiveness: sequestration. Essentially, the parties to the relationship must be kept separate—they must, to the maximum extent possible, be prevented from establishing any kind of relationship. Sometimes the relationship must exist, or already does exist. However, even in such cases, sequestration provides the right policy orientation: the parties must be kept as separate as possible. The ultimate goal is to prevent the antecedent acts between the parties that create favorable states of mind that in turn lead to behavior of partiality. Unlike disclosure, sequestration does work for the precise reason that it interrupts the process that leads to such behavior. If antecedent acts do not occur or are strictly limited, it is much less likely that the parties will form the favorable states of mind that produce behavior of partiality. Thus, it is no surprise that ethicists and commentators are virtually unanimous in their recommendation that health professionals must not be contracted with and compensated directly by teams.

Some ethical problems are difficult; this recommendation is not one of them. There is no satisfactory justification for continuing to structure a model of health care delivery for participants in a violent, dangerous collision sport that knowingly exposes those participants to increased risks of harm flowing from motivated bias and COIs. As the 2016 *Football Players Health Study at Harvard University* puts it, "a system that requires heroic moral and professional judgment in the face of a systemic structural conflict of interest is one that is bound to fail, even if there are individual doctors who manage to negotiate this conflict better than others."[32] Such a system should be abandoned immediately, and a model of care should be instituted that takes care to sequester, to the maximum extent possible, the health professionals charged with the care of players from the sources of compensation for such care. The very fact of such compensation alone brings health professionals and teams (or the NFL as a whole) into some kind of relationship. As physician-bioethicist Howard Brody has noted, "All known ways of paying physicians create temptations to act in ways that fail to serve the patient's health. . . . But we have discovered no way to deliver health care without paying physicians."[33] Yet, again, the policy recommendation here does not require that we live in a utopia where such relationships can always and in every case be eliminated. We can create organizations and entities that sequester and separate the relevant parties to the maximum extent possible. Perhaps the NFL could reorganize and require all teams to pay a certain annual amount into a health professional group not owned or controlled by the NFL. The NFLPA, for example, could contract directly with such a group to administer and provide services for players.

Such a model is not novel—many large employers in the US contract with third-party administrators to structure, deliver, and ultimately pay health professionals for the care their employees and workers require. Indeed, the lack of novelty is ultimately the point—while such arrangements are beset with a host of their own problems, they are somewhat less subject (at a minimum) to the extreme problems of motivated bias and COIs posed by the direct care model to which the NFL and its teams cling.

Conflicts of Interest in College, High School, and Youth Football Organizations

Thus far, the analysis has focused on the COIs and motivated bias problems that attend professional tackle football. But what of the millions of youths and adolescents who play American tackle football?

Beginning with the oldest of these players, American college football nurtures profound COIs.[34] Akin to the NFL, these COIs are mostly structural: health professionals charged with caring for football players are compensated, and in many cases are even directly employed, by the universities that benefit from the participants' play. As Christine M. Baugh and colleagues note, "In the case of college athletes, two main non-clinician stakeholders that could be seen as having an influence on athletes' health related decision-making are the athlete's coach and the school's athletic department, which often serves as a supervisory structure for both the coach and the clinician."[35] The "supervisory structure" is important for making sense of COIs, since it establishes that health professionals charged with caring for players have strong relationships with a third party that has a vested interest in player participation. This dynamic has only become more apparent in the COVID-19 pandemic, in which universities across the US continued to facilitate and encourage tackle football, even while doing so unquestionably posed elevated risk of spreading the disease among the team, the university community (non-athlete students, staff, faculty, etc.), and the towns and cities in which the universities are situated.[36]

The extent of COIs experienced by health professionals and officials among high school and youth football in the US is much more difficult to assess. The governing body for high school football, the National Federation of State High School Associations, updated its guidelines in

2019. These guidelines provide in part that high school associations must assure emergency services coordination with local emergency medical services (EMS), on-site health care services, and health care administration under the auspices of a supervising medical director.[37] To the extent that these health care professionals are compensated by the associations or the teams themselves, the same kinds of structural COIs discussed in this chapter are of concern.

Below the varsity high school level, there is a lack of rigorous studies and likely no data source sufficient to enable researchers to determine whether and the extent to which COIs exist among health professionals charged with caring for participants in American tackle football.

Indeed, on an even more basic level, below the college level, it is quite possible that health professionals are insufficiently available to attend to the health needs of the football players. While leagues and teams sponsoring and paying for health professionals is a public health problem because it poses COIs, an insufficiency of health professionals is also an enormous public health problem. Moreover, several studies call into question the actual sufficiency of medical and health care services in high school.[38] Even more alarming is a 2012 study that found,

- in some public schools, a large number of coaches lacked basic certification in CPR and first aid;
- most school administrators did not have a plan for offering minimal emergency equipment, ice, or water for visiting teams; and
- administrators failed to assure the existence of an emergency action plan or a health professional trained in catastrophic injury management.

Ultimately, the investigators found that seven out of the eight Essential Event Coverage components provided in the American Academy of Pediatrics' "Self-Appraisal Checklist for Health Supervision in Scholastic Athletic Programs" were not addressed by the public schools surveyed in the study.[39]

From an ethical perspective, an inability to ensure basic health care services for children and adolescents playing a violent collision sport is arguably sufficient justification for outright prohibition. Given the certainty of injuries sustained by a vulnerable population, the discharge of a basic responsibility to care for participants onto the youths and families themselves is ethically indefensible. The larger context here reveals the full scope of the ethical problem: either health professionals compensated by teams or leagues are available to care for players, or health professionals are not available at all. In the former case, the population health harm posed by COIs pertains. In the latter case, an even more fundamental population health harm exists: a lack of health professionals sufficient to prevent and care for injuries to players.

×××

COIs are population health harms. This makes identifying and countering them important in whatever context they arise. Historically, COIs have played a critical role in the Manufacture of Doubt, and regulated industries have aggressively pursued relationships with physicians, scientists, nurses, and any other health professionals through whom they can acquire credibility. Unfortunately, COIs generally arise from the relationships we form with others, which makes them extremely difficult to root out and to address. No remedies, short of preventing the relationships from which they emerge, has any solid evidence of effectiveness. In the American tackle football industry, COIs are deeply seeded in the very structure of health care for participants. These structures persist at college and high school levels. Sport reflects the conditions of the society in which it exists, and this is especially true for deep play. In a society that tolerates and even encourages significant COIs in its health care organizations in general, finding the same kind of toleration in a deep play game like American tackle football is unsurprising.

The most effective remedy for the COIs that plague American tackle football is "sequestration": preventing, to the maximum extent possible, the relationships between teams, leagues, and health professionals. While chapter 6 discusses this remedy in more detail, another ethical justification for adopting the policy of sequestration is in preventing the known risks of harm that flow from COIs. This notion of prevention is at the core of the "precautionary principle," which is itself a critical component of the ethical justification for regulating the harms of tackle football via laws and policies. Chapter 5 therefore explains the precautionary principle and why it matters so much for protecting vulnerable groups from public health hazards, including collision sports.

Unreasonable Demands for Proof of
Causation and the Precautionary Principle

This chapter addresses the role of the Precautionary Principle (PP) in ethical and legal issues surrounding collision sports and TBI.[1] Although there are many ways of defining and understanding the PP, the most important idea is that the PP acts as an evidentiary warrant for public health action. The idea of a "warrant" matters because we must know when we are justified in intervening in the name of public health. What kinds and levels of evidence are sufficient to generate such a justification?

As noted in chapter 1, these kinds of questions are at the core of this book. The PP is critical in part because virtually every public health intervention imposes costs. Regulations and public health laws can be especially burdensome. We need some way to array the benefits and the burdens, and to understand what knowledge of the risks of a given exposure justifies public health intervention at the level of laws and policies. The stakes are enormous. If we maintain a very strict standard for the amount and quality of evidence needed to justify public health action, there is an elevated risk of type II errors (false negatives). That is, we will choose not to intervene even in cases where an intervention could prevent or mitigate a serious public health problem. Conversely, if we permit a very loose standard for the amount and quality of evidence needed to justify public health action, there is an elevated risk of type I errors (false positives). That is, we will choose to intervene even in cases where a perceived problem turns out to have little health impact at all. In this latter case, there will be relatively few benefits to be gained from a robust public health response, but there are potentially many burdens imposed via public health laws and policies.

Thus, discerning when and where to draw the line for public health action is critical. And the PP is at the core of this task; it helps us define and specify the warrant for public health action of any kind. It helps a society decide when and where public health action is justified. A basic definition of the PP is "when in doubt about the presence of a hazard, there should be no doubt about its prevention or removal."[2] The term has its origins in environmental health and policy discussions of the 1970s, where the probability of a particular harm was unknown, but the magnitude of the harm, were it to occur, would be immense. The question that gave birth to the idea of the PP was the same faced in thinking about collision sports and TBIs: What level of proof is needed to justify intervening to prevent a public health harm? And what intensity of interventions are justified to counter the risks of a given problem or exposure? The basic definition above offers a rudimentary concept for understanding the PP, but it is inadequate to resolve these difficult questions. It cannot be the case that the mere presence of a hazard justifies any intervention actors could undertake to prevent or remove that hazard. Over 30,000 Americans die in automobile accidents every year, and we do not prohibit driving as a means of preventing these fatalities.

While the PP has benefited from a resurgence of scholarly interest over the last decade, philosopher Daniel Steel's 2015 book is especially useful.[3] In it, he points out that despite efforts to apply and conceptualize the PP since its emergence, "the literature on PP is of a whole . . . disappointingly less than the sum of its parts. Although one finds many interesting insights and proposals related to PP, it is often unclear how these pieces fit together in a logically consistent manner."[4] Steel argues that part of the confusion over the PP is that it is often explicated as a procedural requirement that constrains policymaking, a decision rule "that aims to guide choices among specific . . . policies," or an epistemic rule "that makes claims about how scientific inferences should proceed in light of risks of error."[5] Steel contends that the mistake is to view the PP as any of these in isolation; rather, it is all three.

While Steel argues that all components of the PP are significant, it is the epistemic rule that is most important for ethical policymaking in population health. What do we need to know to warrant a given public health intervention? There is not a unitary answer to this question. We might demand different levels of knowledge before implementing interventions with different intensities. If a public health intervention is especially burdensome, such as imposing a punishing tax, or prohibiting a certain use of private property, society might have reason to require higher standards for the evidence on which the restriction is based. In contrast, public health interventions that do not impose substantial burdens might be justified based on less robust evidence linking an exposure and a harm. And, as noted above, there are enormous stakes in public health for the set point of our epistemic requirements. Therefore, to the extent the PP can help give a justification for relaxing or strengthening the requirements for evidence and knowledge before acting, it is of critical importance.

While the PP may have grown out of international politics in environmental health, its significance is not limited to environmental concerns. In fact, the PP is one of the basic foundations for public health action of any kind. To explain why, it is necessary to consider some features of the evidence bases most relied on to justify public health action. Such evidence frequently derives from epidemiology. Epidemiology is the study of "the distribution . . . and determinants . . . of health-related states and events . . . in specified populations."[6] Like any field, epidemiology is composed of a variety of subfields, with scientists and practitioners specializing in areas such as injury, infectious disease, nutrition, mental and behavioral health, and social factors, to name but a few.

What kinds of evidence does epidemiology produce? To simplify, we can draw a distinction between epidemiology studies that produce evidence of correlation versus those that produce evidence of causation. Traditionally, most epidemiology studies are correlative in nature—they evaluate whether there exists an association between a given exposure and certain health outcomes. Epidemiologists are fully aware that for public health practice and policy, we are most interested in knowing whether a given exposure causes a particular health outcome. Two questions result: First, why do most epidemiologic studies tend to produce evidence of correlation if we would prefer to have evidence of causation? And second, under what circumstances are we justified in inferring a causal relationship from evidence of a correlation?

As to the first question, the reasons why most epidemiology studies tend to produce correlative evidence have to do with ethics and efficiency. One of the best ways of producing evidence of causation is through a randomized controlled trial (RCT). In an RCT, investigators typically set up a control arm and an experimental arm. In the control arm, participants are exposed to a placebo. In the experimental arm, participants are exposed to the variable itself (such as a drug). If the research team is able to control for confounding factors, then the team is justified in inferring that any observed effects in the trial are caused by the variable. RCTs are vastly more complicated than this, and in fact there are many reasons to be concerned with causal inferences in any given RCT.[7] For example, it is often very difficult to eliminate all important confounders, which can bias the results in a number of ways. Nevertheless, there is widespread agreement that a well-designed, methodologically rigorous RCT is a helpful tool in producing evidence of causation between a given exposure and a health outcome.

So, why are RCTs relatively rare in epidemiology? They are rare mostly for reasons of ethics and efficiency. As to the ethical concerns, imagine that we wanted to determine the precise level of benzene exposure that will be toxic to children. We could design an RCT to find out. This would require a control arm and an experimental arm. In the experimental arm, we would intentionally expose children to increasing levels of benzene and monitor for evidence of toxicity. Such an experiment is obviously unethical, since as a rule we do not expose children to toxicants in the interest of determining the precise level at which significant harm ensues. The same ethical concern applies to a great number of the exposures that correlate significantly with health. It is simply not permissible to intentionally expose people and communities, many of whom may be vulnerable in important ways, to known health hazards. Even where the answers to the questions we ask are important from a public health perspective, in epidemiology it is often ethically unacceptable to run RCTs even where doing so would generate helpful evidence of causation.

We can easily apply this ethical concern to collision sports and TBI. We desperately want to know how many TBIs, from what age, and of what severity, are sufficient to cause serious injury and/or long-term neuropathology. It is especially important to know the answer to this question for populations of children and adolescents given their vulnerability. Yet we cannot run an RCT where we intentionally expose children and adolescents to progressive high-impact collisions to learn these answers. Doing so is blatantly unethical. So, we must rely on different kinds of study designs to generate different kinds of evidence in epidemiology.

Moreover, even assuming there were cases where running epidemiologic RCTs would be ethically permissible, they still might be practically and financially impossible. Many health outcomes take many years to develop from the point of exposure. It is not possible to keep participants in an experimental arm of a clinical trial for many years or decades. Too many people would simply leave the trial (called "loss to follow-up"). Moreover, the longer the trial goes on, the more difficult it becomes to control for various confounding factors, since the people in these trials live their lives and will eventually be exposed to all sorts of variables that could bias the results. RCTs also tend to be very expensive to coordinate and maintain, and sustaining one for such a length of time is not financially feasible.

These concerns of ethics and efficiency/cost therefore make it traditionally difficult to run RCTs for many of the various kinds of exposures relevant to health and the study of epidemiology. Before turning to the question of what epidemiologists tend to do instead of running RCTs, it is worth pausing to reflect on one important implication of the general difficulties preventing widespread use of RCTs in epidemiology: if RCTs are generally not possible and indeed are often unethical, it is not reasonable to demand evidence of a kind that can only be generated through RCTs to justify public health action.

To unpack this argument further, we have established that RCTs are frequently impossible to conduct in epidemiology and public health research. We have also established that there are excellent reasons why performing RCTs is impossible—they are inefficient, costly, and most important, are frequently unethical. But if so, then arguing that public health interventions ought not proceed in the absence of causal evidence (of a kind typically generated only by RCTs) is totally unreasonable. Such an argurment is literally equivalent to arguing that public health action of any kind is unjustified! This claim is absurd and should be rejected out of hand.[8] We cannot require standards of evidence for public health action that are literally impossible to meet. If we did, we would lack a justification for public health action of any kind in many situations where RCTs are not possible. Such a scenario is ethically unacceptable since it essentially implies that public health action in general is unjustified. This conclusion is so extreme as to be incompatible with any minimum conception of a just social order.

This chapter will return to this important point, but for now let's briefly consider what kinds of studies epidemiologists typically turn to in the absence of RCTs—and what levels of evidence these different study designs can generate. Although epidemiologists can turn to a wide variety of such designs, arguably the most common are so-called cohort studies. These studies closely track a given cohort to evaluate the extent of an association between a given exposure or exposures and important health outcomes. Cohort studies generate all sorts of useful data; indeed, the bulk of the most important epidemiologic data that researchers have collected and analyzed over the last 40–60 years has come from cohort studies or studies with similar designs. Yet by their nature such studies can only generate correlative evidence, or evidence of a correlation between an exposure and a health outcome. Epidemiologists are well-aware of this, so they turn to two main tasks to address this potential limitation.

First, scientists and researchers attempt to control for confounding variables to the maximum extent possible. The more that such variables can be accounted for and controlled, the more likely it is that a strong association between an exposure and a health outcome represents a real connection rather than a coincidence. Second, epidemiologists invest an enormous amount of resources and work on the subject of causal inference, which asks under what conditions are we justified in inferring causation from evidence of correlation? The scholarly and scientific activity around causal inference has been especially intense over the last 20 years, so much so that "causal inference" is now recognized as a distinct subfield, integrating insights and perspectives from epidemiology, biostatistics, economics, philosophy of science, and policy studies in particular. A number of universities around the world have established "causal inference laboratories" in which cross-disciplinary teams develop different methods for evaluating when and where causal inferences are warranted based on a given analysis. Scientists and researchers typically begin these sorts of inquiries with the Bradford Hill criteria, named after epidemiologist Austin Bradford Hill. These criteria are:

1. Strength of association
2. Consistency
3. Specificity
4. Temporality
5. Biological gradient
6. Plausibility
7. Coherence

8. Experiment
9. Analogy

These are not best understood as true criteria of causation but rather what philosopher of epidemiology Alex Broadbent refers to as aspects of association[9] that in many ways resemble Wittgenstein's family resemblances discussed in chapter 3. Taken together, a correlation that features sufficient levels of most or all of these "aspects" counts as evidence strong enough to justify causal inference. In a 2022 study, investigators Christopher Nowinski and colleagues applied the Bradford Hill criteria to the question of CTE and football.[10] They concluded that "on the fundamental question of the relationship between [repetitive head impact] and CTE, an exploration of the literature through each of Hill's nine viewpoints suggests an extremely high likelihood of a causal relationship. That conclusion is bolstered by the complete absence of evidence for plausible alternative hypotheses."[11] On the first criterion, strength of association (SOA), the authors note that in the Bradford Hill literature, SOAs with an odds ratio of 2:1 or above are generally taken to be strong evidence that justifies causal inference.[12] In three of the four studies with the strongest methodological designs (case-control studies with unexposed controls), the authors note that the odds ratio exceeded 90:1.[13] And even in the fourth study that featured the least-exposed population, the odds ratio exceeded 2:1.[14]

Moreover, epidemiologists are not limited to the Bradford Hill approach, as they use a variety of tools and designs, including but not limited to

- varying outcomes frameworks;
- matching methods;
- standardization;
- propensity scores;
- inverse probability weighting;
- instrumental variables;
- joint effects methods;

- marginal structural modeling;
- causal mediation analysis; and
- sensitivity analysis.

There is one main takeaway here: that most epidemiologic studies generate evidence of correlation is insufficient by itself to justify a claim that a public health intervention is not justified. To be sure, some interventions based on correlative evidence may end up unjustified; but literally countless interventions at local, state, national, and global levels with significant health impact have been undertaken based on correlative evidence. The trick is to distinguish the justified from the unjustified interventions, and the PP turns out to be a critical tool for explaining where we should draw this particular line.

Why? Because the PP provides the ethical justification for intervening on the basis of evidence of correlation. Recall that under Steel's formulation, it is the epistemic component that is most important for practical ethics and policy. The PP helps discern what we need to know in order to justify public health intervention. More specifically, it relaxes the evidentiary warrant for public health action.[15] We do not impose strict standards for evidence of causation to justify at least some public health actions. But the PP is even more important than this because it provides a basic justification for public health action at all. As discussed above, if we imposed stringent requirements for causal evidence between a health hazard and a specific outcome, we would essentially have little public health action of any kind. This is an ethically unacceptable outcome.

While the ethical intolerability of essentially abandoning public health suggests the unreasonableness of demanding strict evidence of causation to justify public health action, the PP definitively slams the door shut on this type of claim. The PP is the philosophical basis for accepting correlative evidence as a sufficient warrant for public health action. Where an identified health hazard poses a substantial risk of significant harm to a large number of people, the PP justifies intervening in the name of public health to prevent the harm from occurring, or at least to mitigate that harm. Public health, as an entire field, rests upon the PP. We do not require strict evidence of causation precisely because the PP permits relaxation of the standards of evidence required to warrant intervention. If we abandoned the PP, very little public health actions of any kind would be justified, which would be utterly disastrous for public and population health (and for health equity).

Before turning to application of the PP to collision sports and TBI, it is worth noting the principal objection to the PP: That it essentially writes a blank check, potentially justifying literally any public health action of any kind regardless of the weakness of the evidence upon which such action is based. This is a real concern. There is no question that some public health actions are not justified based on the quality and/or paucity of the evidence offered in support. Moreover, taken historically, public health actors worldwide have much to answer for. All too often, public health has been wielded in service of colonialist, imperialist, and racist projects. In the US, public health leaders were at the forefront of eugenicist thought and action, and the approximately 75,000 women who experienced involuntary sterilizations did so at the behest and efforts of public health actors.[16] Public health surveillance has often been used to limit services or to coerce BIPOC (Black, Indigenous, or people of color) communities into state-mandated care and congregate living facilities—many health care workers at these facilities maltreated and abused the vulnerable people under their care. On the global scale, public health as an enterprise is literally a creature of colonialism and structural violence. These "unclean hands" mean that setting the boundaries for the fair and equitable scope of public health activities is a critical matter for justice and equity.

Moreover, it is difficult to conceive of a public health intervention that does not in some way impinge on the liberty of the people it impacts. Taxes on cigarettes likely lower rates of smoking but are regressive and therefore also disproportionately impact poor people. A city's use of its eminent domain power to acquire land for a park may require the owner to sell private property at an unchosen time for a sum the owner would not otherwise accept. Seat belt laws require automobile drivers and passengers to buckle up. Thus, virtually all public health interventions infringe on people's liberties. Sometimes these infringements seem relatively minor (e.g., wearing a seat belt). At other times, the infringements are significant (e.g., requiring someone ill with an infectious disease to isolate for an extended period of time). The near certainty that public health action of any kind curbs liberty, combined with the historical tendencies of such action to perpetuate patterns of domination, oppression, and violence give serious weight to the need for limits on public health action. Despite the unquestioned successes of public health and the vast potential for public health to improve health and compress health inequalities, the PP cannot be taken to justify any intervention based on any amount or quality of evidence. In their foundational book on public health law, Lawrence O. Gostin and Lindsay F. Wiley explain that the balance between individual rights or liberties and state action in the name of public health is the basic issue that anchors the entire field.[17] That is, most important questions and issues in public health law turn on how to strike the right balance between infringements on individual liberties and state or collective action needed to implement a crucial public health intervention.

The Precautionary Principle and Tackle Football

It is easiest to parse the limits (and the benefits) of the PP when applying it to a specific case. The analysis of the Manufacture of Doubt shows that one of the most significant issues across social contexts is causation. Determining causation in mass tort litigation involving regulated industries is crucial, but contests over causation are also carried out in the pages of scientific journals, in mass media, and before legislators and regulators in public hearings and sworn testimony. Causation is typically centered because, over time, evidence builds that connects the given exposure and subsequent health harms. But correlation is not causation, and so the question is always whether the exposure to the industrial product (tobacco, pharmaceutical, chemical, etc.) causes the ensuing harm. Moreover, pinning down the precise standard of causation can be very difficult, since health care professionals may have different standards of causation than epidemiologists. And legal standards of causation are distinct from those typically used in health care and in health policy.

But these questions of evidence and causation do not occur in a vacuum. Nor are they "merely" debates in the ivory tower of academia or the cavernous halls of scientific conferences. They have enormous social and political influence precisely because regulated industries have historically used the difficulties involved in proving causation as a powerful wedge in manufacturing doubt. Such use has proved highly effective.

The issue of causation has also become central to debates over the moral and legal permissibility of youth and adolescent participation in American tackle football. There is abundant evidence of significant injuries strongly correlated with tackle football participation, including but not limited to elevated risk of long-term neuropathology, chronic pain, and inflammatory disease. The question is the extent to which participation in tackle football causes these health outcomes. As chapter 3 notes, multiple actors associated with the tackle football industry have emphasized that the evidence of causation is insufficient. Perhaps most notably, Ira Casson, chair of the NFL's Traumatic Brain Injury Committee, made this point the center of his testimony before the US Congress in 2010.[18] In 2018, Jason Chung, Peter Cummings, and Uzma Samadani asserted in a letter for a (non-peer-reviewed) blog that "the pathology and link between head impacts and long-term neurological conditions such as CTE is still unclear, with questions of causation yet to be settled."[19] And the influential 6th Consensus Statement on Concussion in Sport, published in 2023, asserts that "the studies, to date, are methodologically limited because most were not able to examine, or adjust for, many factors that can be associated with the mental health and neurological outcomes of interest."[20] The Statement therefore refuses to endorse a causal link, instead stating, "To establish a clear causal association between sports participation early in life and cognitive impairment or dementia late in life or to quantify that association, future well-designed case–control and cohort studies, that include as many individual risk-modifying and confounding factors as possible, are needed."[21]

These arguments about causation matter greatly for policy. Samadani explicitly makes this move in her book *The Football Decision*.[22] In the absence of sufficient evidence of causation, she argues, the many benefits of participation in youth and adolescent tackle football outweigh the health risks associated with play. (She states that the risk-benefit calculus is less favorable for professional tackle football players than for high school and college players.) In contrast, if the weight of the evidence justifying causal inference grew so strong as to be virtually undeniable by all but the most bad-faith actors, the ethical and legal implications would be relatively clear. That is, assume it became relatively uncontroversial to assert that "participation in youth and tackle football causes significant health harms including but not limited to brain injury, chronic pain, and inflammatory disease among children and adolescents." In the face of such a widely accepted causal link, it seems difficult to argue that it is nevertheless ethical for parents to expose children to these health hazards—especially where the participants themselves are legally unable to consent to the risks of play. As to decisions to expose youths and children to health risks, this book has noted the traditionally wide ethical and legal latitude which parents are afforded. But this latitude is not boundless. Where the causal links are deemed sufficiently clear, many societies, including the US, simply prohibit parents from choosing to expose their children to such harms.

This analysis shows why the debates over causation matter so much in general as to regulated industries and public health harms. But when the affected groups are composed mostly of children and adolescents, the stakes grow even higher. And when the exposure itself is associated with a beloved deep play game like tackle football in the US, those high stakes reach new heights. These questions of causation are therefore not merely academic; they cut to the very heart of the ethical and legal issues surrounding youth and adolescent participation in tackle football. If tackle football causes serious and lifelong health harms to children, the ethical case for precluding parents from exposing their children to such harms becomes quite strong. The tackle football industry is aware of this dynamic, which is why the effectiveness of challenging causation in the Manufacture of Doubt remains an active and vibrant tool in the defense of youth and adolescent participation.

The PP is a critical tool for addressing and attempting to resolve these difficult issues of causation. Why? As noted above, the PP is a key justification for public health action in general. It justifies a kind of epistemic "crediting," a relaxation of the standards of evidence that warrant intervening in the name of public health. If a society required overly strict evidence of causation in the form of an RCT to warrant public health action, that society would have little of it. The consequences of this public health vacuum would be utterly devastating. Although the limits of permissible public health action is a crucial question in public health ethics and law, defining these limits only becomes difficult at the margins. Demanding standards of evidence that essentially neuter public health action of any kind is entirely unethical.

Again, it does not follow from this claim that any kind and amount of evidence is sufficient to justify any particular public health intervention. Rather, what does follow is that in assessing whether public health action is justified regarding a specific exposure-harm link, wielding the claim of "lack of causality" does not end the inquiry.

In social epistemology, or the study of how people come to know social facts, there is a distinction drawn between what knowers can know and the processes by which knowers generate knowledge. It is true that the mere fact of social agreement on the most suitable kinds of such processes does not by itself guarantee the rightness of a perspective. But in the American pragmatic tradition, a variety of theorists agree that coherence, fairness, and equity in process is on the whole more likely to generate accurate knowledge.[23] It follows that when evaluating social contests about (evidence of) causation, if a relevant community of experts develops, evaluates, and then uses a given set of standards to judge the reliability of knowledge produced, then we should at least pay attention. Thus, it is prudent to consider the perspective of the epistemic communities typically charged with deciding whether public health intervention is justified. And what of the body of evidence linking participation in American tackle football to health harms? Does it pass reasonable standards of evidence of the sort accepted by these epistemic communities?

The answer is "yes." In fact, it is not a close call; the body of evidence easily passes the standards needed to justify regulatory intervention. For example, in a 2019 paper in the prominent journal *Neurology*, Zachary O. Binney and Kathleen E. Bachynski offered a lower-bound estimate of the percentage of former NFL players that could be expected to go on to develop CTE. They found the lowest possible estimate to be near 9.6% and thus concluded, "CTE prevalence in this cohort of NFL players is high under most plausible scenarios."[24]

Scientific and public health bodies have begun to incorporate the evidence supporting causal inference between the kinds of repetitive head impacts involved in collision sports and long-term neuropathology. In 2022, the US National Institute of Neurological Disorders and Stroke (NINDS), one of the National Institutes of Health, altered language on its website to note the research, suggesting that CTE is "caused in part by repeated traumatic brain injuries."[25] The CDC has since adopted similar language in its fact sheet on CTE: "The research to date suggests that CTE is caused in part by repeated traumatic brain injuries, including concussions, and repeated hits to the head, called subconcussive head impacts."[26]

Adam M. Finkel and Kevin F. Bieniek note that scientific regulatory communities in the US have historically and consistently used generally accepted risk and evidence paradigms in implementing policy and precautions intended to protect population health.[27] Accordingly, they tracked the general approach used by the US Occupational Safety and Health Administration (OSHA) to estimate the lowest possible risk that a professional tackle football player will develop CTE. Applying OSHA standards, Finkel and Bienek examined a cohort of 17,150 players over the last 45 years, and estimated that "6.4 per thousand to . . . 13 per thousand" players would develop CTE.[28] They observe that these estimates are biased towards the null, which means that the actual risk very likely exceeds the risk-estimate range they offer. (Biasing towards the null is a technique often used in epidemiology to assess risk, since it means that scientists need not be able to specify the actual risk: where all assumptions and parameters are biased towards zero, the actual risk is very likely greater than the range offered in the estimation.) Finkel and Bieniek also note that the conservative risk-estimates they calculate easily exceed the levels of quantified risk at which OSHA typically initiates regulatory, preventive, and protective action.[29]

There are two important points in Finkel and Bieniek's analysis. One is substantive: the available evidence of a link between exposure to tackle football and severe neuropathology like CTE easily surpasses that required to justify a public health intervention. The fact that the intervention Finkel and Bieniek endorse is a regulatory response is also significant from a public health law perspective. The use of law to prevent or ameliorate health harms flowing from products marketed by regulated industries is critical and is the central subject of chapter 6. Recall that a central objective for regulated industries in deploying the Manufacture of Doubt is the creation or perpetuation of a regulatory vacuum. Although regulated industries are not always opposed to governance of their commercial enterprises, intensified legal and regulatory action are often powerfully adverse outcomes for the industries.

The second point is that the weight of the evidence connecting participation in tackle football with serious health harms satisfies the relevant epistemic standards of people whose profession and expertise is entirely focused on discerning the circumstances under which intervention is warranted. To explain this point a bit further, recall the idea that epidemiologists and public health scientists are acutely aware of the difference between correlation and causation. Indeed, where the vast majority of epidemiologic studies are correlative, it would be peculiar if the question of when these kinds of evidence justify causal inferences were not central to the field. As noted earlier in this chapter, epidemiologists and scientists have developed a range of techniques and methods to discern whether a particular case or study merits causal inference. Taken together, this shows that there exist generally accepted standards in the relevant epistemic community for that process of discernment. Anyone charged with making these kinds of assessments is absolutely part of the community of knowers or "discerners." This would include health care professionals of various kinds, athletics officials, university and school administrators, coaches, parents, and players themselves. But it also includes experts whose training and profession depends on making these kinds of assessments day in and day out, for years on end.

In other words, assessing whether evidence of an exposure-harm link warrants intervention is literally what many epidemiologists and virtually all public health regulators do as an ordinary part of their profession. What these communities of expert knowers widely and generally accept as appropriate standards for causal inference and a warrant for action is both valuable and overall is reliable as a justification for intervention. Note that this claim goes to the existence of generally accepted standards in the relevant community of expert knowers. Experts will often disagree on the application of these standards to any given case problem; standards are not formulae that automatically produce results. But there is typically much less dissent within the relevant epistemic communities on the standards to be applied in discerning whether a causal inference and/or public health intervention is justified. "Although problems of evidence and proof are of course significant within the practice of public health, epidemiologic science is unquestionably accepted by participants in that epistemic community as a legitimate basis for inferring causation to a level sufficient to merit public health action."[30]

Finkel and Bieniek's analysis underscores this critical point. Under standards generally accepted by expert risk analysts and public health regulators, the evidence of an exposure-harm link between tackle football and neuropathology is more than sufficient to warrant regulatory intervention. The power of this argument is even more apparent when it is applied to opposing claims. Opponents of stricter limits of or further public health interventions of American tackle football typically argue that the evidence is simply insufficient to justify such actions. They argue that the correlative evidence by itself does not warrant suggested limits, such as bans on participation in tackle football for players under the age of 14. But what evidence would suffice to merit such an intervention? Requiring the kinds of evidence that can only be obtained via an RCT is absurd on its face for the reasons detailed in this chapter. Doing so would be profoundly unethical, especially with youths and children as test participants. We cannot intentionally expose children to repeated collisions to determine the precise point at which injury ensues (and chronic or later-life injuries might not manifest for many years after the study, which is yet another reason RCTs are often infeasible). Moreover, requiring RCT-style evidence before acting in the name of public health is not consistent with the application of the PP. The PP relaxes the evidentiary requirements for intervening in the name of public health, which is why it is foundational to the entire field. Demanding RCT-style evidence flies in the face of the standards for public health action generally accepted by the relevant community of experts who practice such discernment every day.

Experts are often mistaken, of course. This analysis should not be taken as a call for a kind of absolute and technocratic deference to experts. Histories of medicine and public health are replete with cases in which people with lived experience understood their own diseases and impairments in ways that experts would only begin to apprehend much later in time and space. But here again, note the critical distinction between the standards of evidence people might want to apply in discerning whether intervention is justified and what that evidence suggests in any given case. Opponents of regulation and intervention regarding American tackle football are not simply disputing the facts of a given case—they are arguing that the general standards for intervention are mistaken. There is no adequate justification for abandoning the PP as applied to this specific public health problem. Arguing that the long-standing use of the PP is justified when thinking about the standards for clean water or air pollution but not tackle football is a case of special pleading. But it is completely unjustified, since in all the most important ways, regulated industries that market products that expose vulnerable groups to significant risks of serious long-term health hazards ought to be treated alike in deciding when regulation is warranted. At the very least, there should be legitimate reasons for treating tackle football differently than the pharmaceutical or automobile industry, for example. No such reasons exist here.

There is similarly no good reason for demanding the kinds of evidence produced from RCTs when doing so would be practically impossible and likely unethical, especially where we explicitly do not demand such standards as applied to other public health problems. Nonexpert stakeholders have every right to participate in public reason and debate regarding when and under what circumstances public health laws and policies should be used to curtail the health risks of participation in collision sports. It is significantly less reasonable to argue that the very standards to be used in assessing that evidence should essentially determine the application itself. If opponents of intervention had their way in asserting that only strict evidence of causation were sufficient to justify intervention, very few public health actions would be justified.

Moreover, opponents of public health and regulatory action intended to diminish the health harms that youths and adolescents experience as a result of playing tackle football are almost universally quiet on what evidence would warrant further restrictions. If the current body of evidence is insufficient, then what level and type of evidence would justify public health intervention? Any answer that indicates "We need strict evidence of causation such as the kind produced from RCTs" is fallacious for the reasons noted in this chapter. The inference, then, is that the denial of a sufficient warrant for public health (law) actions is essentially intended to preserve the status quo. Such preservation is a principal outcome desired by regulated industries following the Manufacture of Doubt, "through which claims of insufficient causal evidence have been used time and again to forestall any policy action and maintain the status quo."[31]

It is worth noting one additional point about these conflicts over causation in context of collision sports and tackle football in particular: They are almost entirely directed at the health outcome of neuropathology and, in particular, of CTE. To some extent, this is understandable, as CTE is the most severe and frightening of the health harms associated with participation in collision sports. But, as emphasized throughout this book, a full accounting of the health harms posed by collision sports mandates fair consideration of all health hazards with which the activity is strongly associated. No legitimate public health approach excludes illness, injury, and suffering associated with a given exposure simply because a different illness is more severe. A legitimate risk analysis must include all harms associated with the exposure. Doing so is especially important in weighing debates over causation because some of the health hazards associated with tackle football have significantly stronger evidence of causation than does CTE (which does not imply the evidence of causation for the latter is weak in an absolute sense, only that it is relatively weaker than the evidence of causation for other health harms).

For example, participation in tackle football is strongly associated with the development of inflammatory disease and with chronic pain. (These two conditions are highly "comorbid," which simply means that they frequently occur together.) A 2009 study found that arthritis was three times as common in a population of retired NFL players under the age of 60 as in the general population of the same age range.[32] Another study documents that knee injuries of the kind commonly occurring in tackle football make a person four to six times more likely to develop chronic arthritis.[33] Several studies also show that participation in college football is associated with substantially lower health-related quality of life later in life.[34] In 2016 Janet E. Simon and Carrie L. Docherty studied the health-related quality of life of former college athletes, and found the largest difference in the category of "bodily pain" between athletes who had participated in collision sports and athletes who had participated in limited-contact sports.[35] This is consistent with survey data showing that approximately 93% of retired NFL players with a mean age of 48 reported experiencing persistent pain, and 81% of the total population perceiving their pain to be moderate or severe.[36] Moreover, Simon and Docherty also found that former college collision athletes reported significantly higher rates of depression than the comparison group,[37] which matters because depression and pain are also highly comorbid and each can make the other worse.

In any event, there is no serious dispute regarding the causal connection between participation in tackle football and significantly increased likelihood of inflammatory disease and chronic pain (at the least). Moreover, the longer the exposure (i.e., the longer a person plays), the greater the risk of developing these conditions such that, at least at the professional level, there is little question regarding the likelihood of experiencing these illnesses later in life.

×××

The above analysis shows why the evidence documenting associations between participation in tackle football and ensuing health harms is more than sufficient to justify a public health response. The PP provides the needed epistemic warrant. While the PP is not a blank check justifying any public health response to any amount or quality of evidence, it would be absurd to impose strict causal standards for epidemiologic evidence connecting football to health harms. Such a demand is practically impossible and downright unethical in many cases. It ignores the ordinary evidentiary standards that relevant communities of knowledge-makers and experts rely on in their work, and abandoning a commitment to the PP essentially jettisons the justification for public health action in general. Finally, opponents of regulatory and public health interventions for tackle football have consistently failed to specify what evidentiary standards they believe would justify intervention. This failure licenses the inference that perhaps the primary goal of such efforts is to maintain the status quo, that is, to prevent public health and regulatory action.

The fact that this goal is essentially identical to regulated industries' primary aim in using the Manufacture of Doubt is important, because it illustrates why protestations of good faith and good intent are unhelpful. Recall from chapter 4 that the fact that a party might not intend to let relationships motivate bias has little impact on the extent to which a given entanglement does motivate bias. A physician who cultivates deep relationships with pharmaceutical companies is much more likely to change their behavior because of those relationships, regardless of whether they intend to act only in the patient's best interests.

Moreover, as discussed above, the main issue is not whether the evidence of causation is sufficient, but whether the evidence is sufficient to justify public health action. And on this latter point, the PP is always relevant in determining the legitimate expectations society should have of scientific and epidemiologic evidence. As applied to youth and adolescent participation in American tackle football, the body of evidence is more than sufficient to justify public health action. Specifying these interventions is the subject of the final chapter of this book.

6

Policy Recommendations

By ordinary epidemiologic standards, an activity that exposes people to significant risks of TBI, musculoskeletal injury, and inflammatory disease poses a serious health hazard. The gravity of the problem intensifies where the exposure is one that affects a significant number of people, and/or affects especially vulnerable groups. The exposure at issue here checks both of these boxes, as millions of people in North America alone are exposed annually, and youths and adolescents comprise the vast majority of the exposures.

Chapter 5 establishes the ample evidentiary warrant for intervening to alleviate these risks. That is, the weight of the epidemiologic evidence easily surpasses the standards for intervention imposed by application of the precautionary principle. Maintenance of the status quo is essentially a primary goal of the Manufacture of Doubt and is ethically unacceptable given the health risks detailed throughout this book.

However, merely establishing that public health intervention is warranted is insufficient. A variety of such interventions could be applied, ranging from banning participation in collision sports for certain groups or age cohorts to more incremental approaches such as rule changes. And to make matters even more complex, as noted in chapters 3 and 5, some of these so-called interventions are in truth components of the Manufacture of Doubt, as in when the tobacco industry admitted the potential harmfulness of cigarettes as a way of introducing "low-tar" products (that then caused a great deal of harm in the long run).

As applied to American tackle football, Kathleen E. Bachynski and I argued in 2014 that the tackle football industry is pushing a risk frame that suggests that intervening to prevent or minimize the harms of participation is largely a matter of individual agency and resources.[1] Thus, when the inevitable occurs and a youth or adolescent is injured, including seriously, it is always a failure of individual responsibility (i.e., a player or players' fault for not following "safety rules," insufficient care taken by the referees, an equipment failure, or perhaps even the responsibility of an individual coach). The possibility that an ethically unacceptable risk of serious harm inheres in the nature of the activity by virtue of it being a collision sport is a risk frame the tackle football industry wants to avoid at all costs.

> A risk frame which began from the premise that, even if the precise odds ratios remain to be calculated, (1) some significant level of risk attends play, and continued with the additional premise that (2) rule and technical changes are unlikely to reduce this risk substantially, would likely produce a very different public discourse among families and communities regarding the acceptability of the risk for children and adolescents.[2]

Unsurprisingly, shifting the risk frame from the activity or product of the regulated industry itself to downstream users is a technique in the Manufacture of Doubt. To understand why this technique is favored, we need to return to the primary goals of those industries which use the Manufacture of Doubt. Specifically, one such goal is sustaining, fueling, and/or advancing a policy or regulatory vacuum. Although chapters 2 and 3 discuss this objective at length, the key here is perceiving that the goal operates on the level of policy and regulation. The aim is to avoid the creation of laws, policies, or other governance structures that interfere with the production, marketing, and sale of the product under scrutiny.

But if laws and policies were not powerful tools for addressing health hazards, regulated industries would not fight so hard to prevent their creation or enhancement. In other words, regulated industries have long recognized what epidemiology has begun to show definitively: law is a powerful social determinant of health.[3] This basic idea is at the core of what is known as "public health law." Lawrence O. Gostin and Lindsay F. Wiley define public health law as "the study of the legal powers and duties of the state to assure the conditions for people to be healthy (to identify, prevent, and ameliorate risks in to health in the population) and the limitations on the power of the state to constrain the autonomy, privacy, liberty, proprietary, or other legally protected interests of individuals for the common good."[4]

Tracking the first part of this definition, societies can use laws in ways that "assure the conditions for people to be healthy." Gostin and Wiley note, "Law and policy tools can facilitate many public health interventions, such as ensuring access to education, economic opportunity, healthy food, safe housing, and medical care; facilitating healthier behavior choices; reducing environmental pollution; and creating health-promoting built environments."[5] The COVID-19 pandemic has also demonstrated, beyond any doubt, the ways that different laws and policies can slow transmission and therein affect not only the overall course of the pandemic in any given area but also its distribution (i.e., which communities experience greater or lesser pandemic impact). This reveals an important aspect of public health law to which this chapter will return: public health law has powerful distributive effects, which mean it can serve as a tool for the advancement of health equity. Gostin and Wiley explicitly tie this equity focus to their definition of public health law, observing that consistency with the ideals of justice is its ethical basis.

The idea that laws and policies can strongly influence health outcomes seems uncontroversial, especially when the analysis includes laws and policies that are not enacted or implemented (which can occur for many reasons, but which is a chief objective of the Manufacture of Doubt). But public health law is not simply one social determinant of health among many: it is properly ranked among the most significant factors that determine both overall population health and its distribution. Gostin and Wiley state, "Of the ten great public health achievements in the twentieth century, all were realized, at least in part, through law reform or litigation (e.g., vaccination mandates; workplace, food, and motor safety standards; cigarette taxes and smoke-free laws; and programs to ensure access to prenatal and pediatric medical care and nutrition)."[6]

Ultimately, there is overwhelming evidence that laws and policies are powerful social determinants of health. This basic observation has sprouted new directions in public health law research, many of which treat law as an epidemiologic exposure like any other. By virtue of living in society, all of us, including children, are exposed to health-promoting (i.e., recreational spaces, safe housing, quality education, access to nutritious food, etc.) and health-damaging (i.e., lead, wildfire smoke, unsafe housing, discrimination and racism) factors. While we are not used to thinking of laws and policies as such an exposure, the epidemiology makes perfectly clear that there is no good reason to avoid doing so. Laws and policies have a powerful impact on health and its distribution and should therefore be regarded and studied just as any epidemiologic exposure. The nascent field of legal epidemiology has emerged to answer this call and produce evidence documenting the impact of laws and policies on important population health metrics.[7]

Laws are not exclusively health-promoting, of course. It takes little imagination to consider unjust or harmful laws that actively diminish a person or an entire community's health. Laws permitting chattel slavery and/or authorizing the persecution and attempted genocide of Indigenous peoples in the US are obvious examples of such deleterious laws, the effects of which continue to the present.[8] And laws are no different from any other kind of health intervention, in the sense that even the best of intentions do not guarantee positive health impact. Some health interventions work poorly or not at all, and for all their power, laws enjoy no inherent advantage in the likelihood that they will improve health and compress health inequalities.

Indeed, there are already public health laws in force in the US that attempt to address TBI and other health harms that attend participation in collision sports. The most common such laws are screening and reporting laws that mandate youth, adolescent, and college athletes who are experiencing symptoms of a TBI arising from play receive an adequate screening and have their health condition documented and reported to the appropriate authorities.[9] While such laws are an important step in establishing better public health law governance over collision sports among youths and adolescents, they nevertheless are subject to a number of drawbacks that limit their potential health impact. First, such laws only come into effect once a participant has experienced or is experiencing symptoms of a TBI. They therefore do little to advance the crucial public health goal of prevention. It is preferable to prevent TBI and other injuries associated with collision sports from occurring than to treat them once they have occurred. Second, screening and mandatory reporting requirements are part and parcel of what is known as "public health surveillance." There are many kinds of public health surveillance, including infectious disease surveillance that has taken on particular importance during the COVID-19 pandemic. Such infectious disease surveillance is also important for youth and adolescent sports, given the evidence that participation in such activities has a marked impact on community spread.[10] Likewise, injury surveillance is critically important for youth and adolescent collision sports, and it forms a cornerstone of good public health and health care practice for participants.

Yet while public health surveillance is essential for virtually any activity that exposes participants to significant risks, in isolation it is a poor health intervention. The value of surveillance is that it can help officials, families, and communities identify important health risks and then take all steps needed to prevent or minimize those risks. In the absence of such further steps, simply identifying injuries when they occur produces little positive health impact. Effective public health action often depends on good surveillance practices, but good surveillance practices alone do not constitute effective public health action. At the present, there is no good evidence that mandatory TBI reporting laws have positive health impact, although there is evidence that they have some effect on the primary purpose to which they were put: to increase the reporting of TBIs in youth and adolescent collision sports.[11]

The point of the above is not to derogate public health law approaches focused on injury surveillance. Such surveillance serves an important function, and insofar as it enhances community ability to perceive injuries when they occur and implement interventions to protect youths and adolescents after the injury occurs, they are worthwhile. Rather, the following section seeks to build off the foundation of surveillance. Public health laws are too powerful an intervention to limit solely to governance and promotion of injury surveillance. They can do so much more, and the following section explains how.

×××

Public health laws and policies are fundamentally normative. That is, we cannot simply judge the rightness of laws and policies based on whether they are effective. Laws can be highly effective for a given purpose and still be extremely unjust and immoral. The history of public health in the West is filled with examples of laws promulgated in the service of terrible ends, including but not limited to racist, sexist, and eugenicist objectives. Indeed, Western public health is in many important ways a colonial project, with all the myriad sins and injustices that accompany colonialism.

While organized and collective public health action unquestionably has the potential to accomplish much in advancing human health and compressing health inequalities, it has all too frequently fallen far short. This gap is why it is so important to fuse a call for public health law interventions with a robust ethical foundation. Such a commitment alone is no guarantee that a prescribed legal or policy intervention passes ethical muster, but it can act as an important safeguard in avoiding the tendency of public health action to perpetuate structural violence rather than ameliorate it.

As noted above, Gostin and Wiley urge that public health law must satisfy the demands of social justice to be considered ethical. This chapter follows Gostin and Wiley in embracing a commitment to social justice as an ethical touchstone for its legal and policy interventions. Social justice has many different formulations and conceptions; this chapter adopts the model developed by Madison Powers and Ruth Faden.[12]

Powers and Faden's Model of Social Justice

Powers and Faden's model of social justice is complex. Going through it in painstaking detail would detract from the goals of this chapter. Yet, social justice is too important of a concept to leave completely undefined. Doing so risks reducing it to the status of a slogan rather than a robust ethical framework that can guide law and policy.

Regardless of the complexity, key features of Powers and Faden's model can be sketched here as a means of offering needed ethical guidance for public health law. The model is based on the idea of "health sufficiency," the idea that everyone requires access to sufficient measures of the resources needed to live a flourishing life. Powers and Faden term these resources the "six essential dimensions of well-being":

1. Personal security from harm
2. The development of reasoning capacities
3. Respect of/from others
4. The capacity to form personal attachments
5. Health
6. Self-determination

Ethically optimal policies should focus on the factors that tend to drive entire communities below sufficient measures of one or more of these essential dimensions of well-being. In turn, the most culpable factors that drive such insufficiencies are those that cause "densely-woven patterns of disadvantage."[13] A community that experiences such patterns of disadvantage tends to experience clusters of other social disadvantage, all at the same time.[14] Thus a community whose members disproportionately experience low socioeconomic position also tend to experience low educational attainment. Such community members are also more likely to live in unsafe housing, lack access to safe recreation spaces, and be exposed to violence, discrimination, and racism. This "compound" disadvantage is an aggregate phenomenon and will not be true of every individual in a given community. But at the community level, it holds uncomfortably well in the US.

From a social justice perspective, laws and policies should prioritize the factors that drive compound or "densely-woven patterns of" disadvantage.[15] The factors that are responsible for these patterns are the same problems that create multiple insufficiencies in the essential dimensions of well-being for some communities. What are some such factors?

At one level, the factors that fuel such insufficiencies are what has been referred to as the social determinants of health. Important social determinants include resources like access to high-quality education, early childhood development, safe recreational opportunities, safe and secure housing, food security, access to safe and affordable transportation, protection from violence and discrimination, and socioeconomic position (SEP). SEP is one of the most powerful predictors of health, both across entire populations and within them, although it is a compound variable that includes a number of factors that themselves exert discrete health impact.[16]

However, as important as it is to name and identify these social determinants of health, they are not generally root causes of densely-woven patterns of disadvantage. The key word here is "patterns" because these social determinants are not self-determining; that is, the fact that safe housing is a powerful determinant of health does not explain why some communities enjoy vastly superior access to safe housing than others. In order to explain densely-woven patterns of disadvantage, we need an account of the variables and factors that explain the incredibly unequal access to important social determinants of health. What are some such factors?

Although here the answer is more complicated, the factors that explain unequal access to critical social determinants are structural forces that closely track historical patterns of domination, oppression, and subordination. As noted in chapter 1, these patterns are characteristic of structural violence; the connections between injustice and structural violence is part of what makes a commitment to social justice in public health law and policy so significant. Social justice is thus a key normative foundation for humane and moral public health laws and policies.

One final point about Powers and Faden's model of social justice is relevant: the framework is what is known as a "twin aims" approach.[17] A twin aims approach is one in which interventions seek to maximize both (1) overall population health and (2) the compression of existing health inequalities. Although a full discussion is unhelpful here, there is no shortage of examples of public health policies that improve overall health at the same time they expand health inequalities. For example, since 1990 the US has lowered the incidence and prevalence of smoking, which is unquestionably good for overall population health. But inequalities in smoking have dramatically increased in the same time period, which is ethically problematic. Although this does not necessarily mean that a particular public health law or policy that only accomplishes one of the two aims is ethically unacceptable, it does suggest that such an intervention is ethically suboptimal. We should prioritize approaches that promise both to improve overall population health and to compress health inequalities. This prioritization is what a commitment to the twin aims of social justice in health entails.

To bring this analysis back to the level of policy guidance, the key takeaway points are:

1. Ethically optimal public health policies are those that target the densely-woven patterns of disadvantage that are most responsible for creating multiple insufficiencies in the essential dimensions of well-being.
2. The factors that are most responsible for driving such patterns are structural forces like racism, uncontrolled rent and profit-seeking, and stigma.

3. These structural forces are deeply linked to historical constellations of domination, oppression, and subordination, which makes the general concept of "structural violence" introduced in chapter 1 so important for ethical policymaking.

The remainder of this chapter applies this social justice framework to four core policy recommendations for alleviating the public health harms caused by collision sports in youth and adolescent populations.

Policy Recommendation #1: Ban Tackling for Participants under the Age of 14

Youths and adolescents under the age of 14 should be prohibited from engaging in tackling or collisions of similar force in any sanctioned league, practice, or game of American football.

Calls to ban tackling among youths and adolescents are not novel. As noted earlier in the book, several states have introduced bills to enact such a ban, although to date none have yet become law. The justification for implementing this prohibition is strong from both epidemiologic and ethical perspectives.

Public health justification

Abundant evidence from neurology, kinesiology, and injury epidemiology shows why youths and younger adolescents are particularly vulnerable to injuries resulting from collision sports. In 2018, the *Concussion Legacy Foundation* issued a white paper laying out the public health justification for banning tackle football for participants under the age of 14.[18] First, from a neurological perspective, the period between roughly 8–13 years of age is critical for brain development in at least three areas:

1. White matter development (when nerve cells become myelinated, which protects the cells and increases the speed of communication between them)

2. Grey matter development (when brain structures controlling memory and emotion peak)

3. Peak cerebral blood flow (when blood flow to the cerebrum peaks, "reflecting the growth and maturation of many regions of the brain")[19]

Second, adolescents under the age of 14 have insufficiently developed neck muscles in proportion to the size and weight of their head (which is actually larger, relative to their body weight, than for adults).[20] This "Bobblehead Effect" is the principal reason why, despite adolescents being significantly slower and smaller than adults, studies show the force of the collisions in youth and adolescent football is consistent with the force documented among older adolescents and even among adults.[21]

Third, the White Paper reminds that the neurological harms are not etiologically limited to diagnosed or even undiagnosed concussions. Rather, subconcussive impacts are strongly associated with all manner of adverse and pathological neurological changes and are therefore also critical in assessing the known risks.[22]

These considerations have led governing bodies for other youth and adolescent sports to prohibit play that facilitates collisions and/or head impacts. Thus youth hockey leagues in both Canada and the US have banned bodychecking; and there is documented evidence that these bans have reduced TBIs.[23] Youth soccer associations in the US in 2015 and in the UK in 2020 have banned or restricted heading, both because of the repeated impacts involved in practicing heading and because of the collisions that ensue during aerial play. In short, there is ample justification for banning tackling in American football for participants below the age of 14. (As to why the age of 14 and whether such a cut-off is a weakness is addressed below under Objection #4.)

There is no serious dispute regarding the risks and health hazards noted above. There is, of course, vigorous debate regarding the extent to which such hazards result in long-term, chronic health conditions for participants. But even the NFL has acknowledged the health risks for youth and adolescent participants in particular. As chapter 2 notes, such concessions are themselves a key part of the Manufacture of Doubt. In the face of overwhelming epidemiologic evidence linking exposure and harm, "blanket denials are not credible."[24] Again, the tobacco industry advanced this particular technique in the Manufacture of Doubt, where acknowledging health harms associated with the use of the product in question are "wrapped in a package of accommodation and reasonableness."[25] This package is then attached to new safety initiatives and harm reduction initiatives as a way of building or sustaining a political and regulatory vacuum.

Nevertheless, in the absence of a credible basis for disputing the evidence linking tackling for players under the age of 14 to serious health hazards, the opposition to banning tackling in this cohort has typically proceeded on policy and ethical grounds. The arguments often revolve around the benefits of preserving the status quo and/or liberty/parental autonomy interests justifying the inclusion of tackling.

Ethical justification

From an ethical perspective, we'll look at issues of parental liberty and disability ethics. There are strong parental liberty traditions in the West, aspects of which are carved especially deeply into the legal architecture of the US.[26] In the realm of medical and health care in particular, parents are legally authorized as surrogates who, in most states, have ultimate authority to make decisions for pediatric patients. While latitude for parental liberty or autonomy is traditionally significant in Anglo-American law, it is neither bought cheaply nor is it boundless. Family historian Steven Mintz points out that even while nineteenth-century social changes emphasized individual responsibility within the family, "it was, paradoxically, during this period that reformers and local governments, eager to rectify parental failures, acquired new authority to act in loco parentis."[27] The tension between the scope of domestic authority within families and the collective obligations to intervene for the sake of child welfare is a constant feature in US history, although the balance and outcomes have shifted across time, place, and community.

Despite the complexity of family law historically, traditionally "parents enjoyed wide discretionary authority over the details of their children's upbringing."[28] Yet, in the contemporary US, Mintz argues that family law is characterized by a "growing sensitivity on the part of courts and legislatures toward the individual, even when family privacy is at stake."[29]

From a disability history perspective in particular, the confidence in parental motivations and capacity to act in their children's best interests has not always been rewarded. The dominance of ableism in the modern West may explain part of this observation—that even parents who intend to help their children may end up reproducing ableist norms in ways that result in harm to children. For example, standard care for children born with talipes equinovarus (clubfoot) had long been repeated surgeries through youth and adolescence to "correct" the body form. The outcomes for these surgeries were often unfavorable, and pain was a common result; today, the majority view is that this form of intervention caused more harms than benefits.[30] We need not presume any ill intent from parents; the normalizing power of ableism and medicalization framed a child's impairment in ways that rendered the contemporaneous standard-of-care (repeated surgical intervention) an acceptable decision.

In essence, the issue of parental liberty or autonomy is one of the central ethical issues underpinning the entire controversy regarding collision sports and youth/adolescent injury. As noted in chapter 1, the key question is: To what extent should parents be permitted to expose their children to risk of harm or injury? We permit parents to do so in many different contexts in US society. Are the dangers of American tackle football so serious that they merit limiting parental authority to make decisions on behalf of their children? And what criteria serve to distinguish the list of risky activities for which parents may enroll their children from those for which society has circumscribed that authority?

These are difficult, complex questions that merit careful attention. However, in the case of American tackle football, for youths under the age of 14, no intricate ethical analysis is necessary. There are almost no conceivable benefits obtainable from playing American tackle football that do not also attend flag football or other forms of football that remove collisions from permitted play. To be clear, the benefits of participation in sport should not be underestimated and may include a variety of positive outcomes. But it remains decidedly unclear why repeated high-speed collisions are needed to obtain any of these benefits. Moreover, given the serious risk of injury and potentially chronic and long-term health harms that attend participation in collision sports, the ethical case in favor of capturing those benefits while drastically reducing the probability of potentially significant harm is decisive. Consider, for example, the famous federal judge Learned Hand's mid-twentieth century calculus for negligence under the law. In the 1947 case of *United States v. Carroll Towing*,[31] Hand suggested that there was a relationship between the burden of taking necessary precautions, the probability of harm, and the gravity of loss; and Hand said that negligence exists when B is less than P multiplied by L (in equation form: $B < PL$), where B is the burden of acting in a way that would have prevented the injury, P is the probability of the harm occurring, and L is the magnitude of the harm were it to occur.

Thus, where a property owner could have easily fixed the pavement in front of their establishment (a small burden, B) and the probability of a person tripping and injuring themselves (P) is high, then even if the harm were only moderately severe (L), negligence has occurred. Although Hand's calculus is simplistic, the point is simply to suggest the existence of a relationship between the three variables. In the case of American tackle football for players under the age of 14, the burden is relatively low to play football without collisions or to play a different sport with much lower risk, the probability of harm occurring is sufficiently high, and the magnitude of loss (harm) is considerably high. Therefore, under this analysis, negligence exists.

(The evidence in support of the probability of harm being sufficiently high in the case of American tackle football has been discussed at length in chapter 5. The weight of this evidence without question justifies a public health intervention, which implies a sufficiency of the evidence regarding risk of harm. That is, if the evidence regarding risk of harm to youths and adolescents were insufficient to justify public health action, it seems unlikely we could declare the probability of harm sufficiently high to charge negligence in the absence of public health action. There is a logical connection between these two positions.)

Although this issue is complex, there is no doubt that, both ethically and legally, in US law there is a sphere within which parents are permitted to make decisions that expose their children to risks of harm. There is also a sphere within which parents are proscribed from making decisions that expose their children to risks of harm. The crux of the ethical issue here is discerning where American tackle football lies within these spheres. Given the weight of the evidence regarding the probability of the harm occurring and the magnitude of that harm were it to occur, there is sound ethical basis for concluding that such participation lies beyond the boundaries of a permissible exercise of parental autonomy.

Moreover, given this book's focus on the "birds-eye view" of public and population health,[32] such decisions cannot be framed solely as an individual choice that a specific set of parents might make on behalf of a specific child. Rather, given the millions of youths and adolescents participating or intending to participate in American tackle football, the ethical question here is one that is best seen as a policy determination that applies to a significant (and vulnerable) population. For population health ethics questions, values that are properties of individuals such as "autonomy" are not necessarily best-suited to weighing owed obligations and the boundaries of permissible conduct for relatively large groups. Rather, ethical concepts rooted in populations and groups, such as "justice," are much more appropriate primary frameworks.

Recall that the health sufficiency model of social justice described above suggests a priority on factors that drive "densely-woven patterns of disadvantage." In addition, to be ethically optimal, policy interventions ought to both improve the overall health of the population of interest and compress existing health inequalities.

Regarding webs of disadvantage, the harms to which youths and adolescents are exposed in American tackle football can become chronic and affect them across the life span. This is true both of neurological and nonneurological injury and illness (such as pain and inflammatory disease). Moreover, these harms must be considered in proper social context; in the US, the harms are magnified because of the relative lack of social policies and resources designed to assist sick people, families, and caregivers. Thus, in his seminal 1996 book on TBI, William J. Winslade argued for a prohibition on boxing, but not solely because of the inherent risks of the sport.[33] Rather, he argued that in a society that all-but-abandons serious investment in rehabilitation, long-term care, and disability supports, the adverse impact of boxing on the participants, their families, and communities was ethically unacceptable.

Thus, the magnitude of the harm is not solely or even mostly a function of the intrinsic properties of the injuries and illnesses associated with participation in American tackle football. Rather, a society like the US that provides precious little social and collective assistance to chronically ill people, their families, and communities will intensify the disadvantages of living with the sequelae of American tackle football in far-reaching and potentially lifelong ways. This point is crucial since it embodies the social model of disability at the core of disability ethics: the extent to which an impairment is disabling turns much less on any intrinsic property of the impairment and much more on the social supports, policies, resources, and accommodations made available to the impaired person.

In addition, neither experiences of nor responsibilities for caring for people with serious neurological, inflammatory, and musculoskeletal illness are equally distributed. People of color are consistently more likely to experience TBI and are more likely to have worse outcomes from TBI than white people.[34] These same racial inequalities have been documented for so-called mild TBI, TBI among children, and TBI among older adults.[35] Moreover, Einat K. Brenner and colleagues noted abundant evidence of differential care for racial and ethnic minorities experiencing TBI, including rehabilitation and long-term care for depression and other mental health problems. "Taken together, this demonstrates that minority groups are sustaining head injuries at higher rates than majority individuals, yet they report less effective medical care from professionals and suffer more extreme consequences of injury, which could have downstream consequences for vocational outcome and quality of life."[36] There are also significant racial inequalities in the prevalence of chronic pain in the US.[37]

Recall that the twin aims approach to social justice requires that policies compress existing health inequalities. Continuing to permit youths under the age of 14 to play American tackle football is extremely likely to expand racial inequalities in both neurological injury and illness and the inflammatory and pain-centric conditions that so often attend participation in collision sports. These inequalities persist across the life span and in a society with a dysfunctional and often entirely absent social safety net, where the enormous costs of caring for people with significant chronic illness will be borne by the families and communities least-resourced to shoulder the burden.[38]

Ultimately, there seems little way to promote participation in American tackle football for youths under the age of 14 that satisfies basic mandates of social justice. Limiting parental autonomy by eliminating tackling for this age cohort is justified by a commitment to social justice in protecting this vulnerable population.

Policy Recommendation #2: Mandate Minimally Sufficient Health Care Services/Professionals

A minimally sufficient level of health care services must be provided for all full-contact sessions in which youths and adolescents participate in American tackle football.

Within the American tackle football industry, the custom has been for health care services that attend play to be sponsored and provided by the individual teams themselves. This is certainly the traditional model within professional, college, and at least some high school tackle football leagues. Among youths and adolescents, the extent to which teams sponsor health care services is less clear. On this point, reliable and comprehensive data is lacking; but it is certain that not all leagues or teams even sponsor or provide health care services for participants. This latter situation is ethically unacceptable. Given the health hazards involved in playing tackle football, teams and leagues that cannot offer minimally sufficient health care services do not have any ethical path to convening and sponsoring tackle football for youths and adolescents.

There are many different ways of interpreting the requirement in the policy recommendation that a "minimally sufficient level" of health care services must be provided to all participants regardless of age or level of play. It should be noted that "none" or "zero" will never qualify as minimally sufficient. If a full-contact session—either practice, game, or any other period—is to be held, there must be some (nonzero) services available to participants. This requirement implies a minimally sufficient level of health care professionals are available to provide such services (it is difficult to imagine how a team could meet the standards required for minimally sufficient services absent providing access to a minimally sufficient number of health care professionals).

For example, in 2021 California enacted the California Youth Football Act.[39] Among other provisions, this Act requires the presence of a minimum of one certified emergency medical technician, state-licensed paramedic, or higher-level licensed medical professional during all preseason, regular season, and postseason tackle football games. While this is an important example of the use of a public health law intervention to reduce harms associated with tackle football, note that its requirements do not extend to practice sessions.

To be sure, part of the issue regarding the inadequacy of basic health care services for participants in American tackle football is the underlying problem of inadequate access to health care services and health care professionals in a wide variety of communities. Rural areas are especially likely to experience deficiencies in such access. For example, the US Health Resources & Service Administration notes widespread shortages in access to primary care professionals, with particular gaps in rural areas (almost 66% of such shortages occur in rural areas).[40] Similarly, for mental and behavioral health professionals, almost 61% of shortages in access are concentrated in rural areas.[41] While there is insufficient national data on access to other forms of specialty care important to collision sports injuries, such as sports medicine and neurology, studies in general show similarly insufficient access to most health care specialties, especially in rural areas.[42]

These shortages in health care professionals have implications for American tackle football and other collision sports teams located in areas that experience such shortages. Where a given area experiences general shortages, it is much more likely that youth sports teams and leagues will also experience difficulties in providing minimally sufficient access to health care professionals and health care services. Collision sports teams and leagues did not create these structural shortages in the health care workforce and in access problems and likely have limited to no power to improve the situation.

There is thus a sense in which it seems unfair to prohibit American tackle football and/or collision sports where minimally sufficient access to health care services cannot be guaranteed for participants. Such a prohibition might also intensify inequalities in participation between more affluent communities that are better able to ensure minimally sufficient access to health care services and the least well-off areas and communities already laboring under health care shortages. Although these objections will be addressed in detail below, for now, the basic point is the same: given the risks of injury and death that attend collision sports, it is simply unconscionable for youths and adolescents to experience such risks without access to the basic health care services that could save lives and reduce the scope of injury. Although this particular problem is not of the tackle football industry's making, it must share the burden precisely because the industry exposes children to serious risks of long-term harm.

At higher levels of play in which organizations, leagues, and teams enjoy more resources, the equity concerns above are less forceful. Ultimately, American tackle football exposes those who play it to elevated and significant risks of long-term health harms. The magnitude of these risks easily warrants public health interventions. To the extent that we permit youths and adolescents to play it at all, knowingly exposing such vulnerable people to serious health harms without the provision of minimally sufficient health care services is ethically intolerable. This is what is known in law and ethics as a "bright-line" test—it is objective, easily understandable, and can be applied in a relatively clear and straightforward manner.[43] If minimally sufficient health care services cannot be guaranteed, youths and adolescents cannot play league-sponsored, organized tackle football.

Policy Recommendation #3A: Mandate Evidence-Based Conflict-of-Interest Policies for Health Care Professionals Involved in Youth and Adolescent Football

Governing bodies for youth and adolescent tackle football should implement a strategy of sequestration between health care professionals and team or governance officials.

Policy Recommendation #3B: Mandate Evidence-Based Conflict-of-Interest Policies for Academic Experts

Academics and university professors should implement a strategy of sequestration between themselves and the American tackle football industry.

Analysis of Policy Recommendation #3A

Chapter 4 explains how and why conflicts of interests (COIs) are a core component of regulated industries' efforts to manufacture doubt. Where deep entanglements between health professionals, scientists, and regulated industries are tolerated, the effects of those COIs in facilitating the Manufacture of Doubt and ensuing population health harms are well-documented. Scholars have even developed the concept of "commercial determinants of health" to capture the impact of COIs on health outcomes.[44]

That deep relationships between health care professionals, scientists, and public health officials are widely tolerated is ethically unacceptable. All stakeholders engaged in the promotion and governance of American tackle football for youths and adolescents should immediately endorse evidence-based COI policies focused on the principle of sequestration. As chapter 4 notes, sequestration is generally defined as a policy by which parties are prevented from establishing any kind of relationship. The ethical problems and health harms that flow from motivated bias and COIs begin when parties enter into a relationship; therefore the only remedy that has been shown to be effective is the elimination of those relationships.

There is much to unpack regarding how a policy initiative focused on sequestration might work. First, it is important to note that social practices in general are constituted by all sorts of prior and existing relationships. Some of these are difficult if not impossible to disentangle or eliminate. This basic fact implies that full sequestration may be unfeasible in some circumstances and that its implementation could present significant practical problems.

These points are legitimate, but the response is that the practical difficulties with implementing a COI policy based on sequestration does not somehow make other approaches magically effective. The evidence is clear that alternative approaches to COIs based on notions of "management" and "disclosure" are ineffective at best and may actually have perverse effects.[45] If as moral agents we wish to eliminate or at least reduce the impact of COIs and the harms to which they expose youths and adolescents that play American football, we have no choice other than to seek implementation of COI policies based on sequestration.

Moreover, sequestration is a guiding strategy for real-world COI policy. It does not follow that full sequestration must always be achieved in every conceivable instance where the policy is applied. Rather, sequestration is best seen as the goal and an orientation to which all initiatives, processes, and actions taken in advancing the policy should be targeted. The goal is, to the maximum extent possible, to sequester especially health care professionals charged with caring for sick and injured players from the parties and agents who have interests that do not always align with the safety and well-being of the participants.

As noted in chapter 4, full sequestration may be impossible for the simple fact that health care professionals ought to be reimbursed for the services they provide. The financial relationship that arises out of this basic requirement is impossible to avoid save in cases where charity or pro bono care is provided. Yet, centering sequestration as an orientation and a policy objective still offers clues and frameworks for how health care professionals can care for participants in youth and adolescent football in ways that minimize the risks and effects of motivated bias.

Ethically, health care professionals such as athletic trainers, nurses, and physicians must be available to care for participants injured via participation in collision sports. But this basic requirement does not imply that all arrangements for the provision of such care are ethically sufficient. Quite the contrary, the custom by which health care professionals are sponsored and reimbursed directly by the teams and leagues themselves intensifies relationships between those professionals and parties who historically have not always prioritized the safety and well-being of participants over competing interests. Since at least the 1970s, scholars and advocates have consistently urged the tackle football industry to change or alter this so-called direct care or direct reimbursement model. To the extent that attempts to "manage" or minimize COIs and motivated bias (regarding health care professionals and American tackle football) do not begin by rejecting the direct care model, they are simply not evidence-based and are likely to intensify the harms to which youths and adolescents are exposed.

What would an evidence-based COI policy that prioritizes sequestration look like? One mechanism that has been proposed is using a third-party administrator that can direct reimbursement for care.[46] Under this mode, individual teams in a league would all make payments to a centralized committee or body. The committee itself would structure health care delivery and reimbursement, thereby minimizing, to the maximum extent possible, direct relationships between the league, teams, and team officials and health care professionals providing services for participants. The notion of using third-party administrators in health care delivery and financing is nothing new in the US; indeed, this is the point. This model arose in part because of the widespread dissatisfaction with direct care models, as described in detail in chapter 4.

Nor is the third-party administrator model free from problems. The most obvious is that the bargaining and economic power wielded by the administrator can be used in ways that are detrimental to sick and injured people. Third-party administrators can also form relationships with other parties, including and especially client relationships with the parties that pay them. Regulations and governance for these relationships will likely also be needed. But, in the end, as noted above, there is simply no way to avoid completely the need to reimburse health care professionals for the services they provide. And there is no ethical way to avoid completely utilizing the services of health care professionals for youths and adolescents participating in an activity as dangerous as tackle football.

Insofar as adolescents age 14 and over participate in American tackle football, they will require health care services to prevent, treat, and assist with rehabilitation of the injuries commonly and uncommonly associated with such participation. The professionals rendering these services must be reimbursed. Such reimbursement is itself a form of exchange that can and does lead to motivated bias and COIs. In addition, health care officials are customarily sponsored, paid, and/or even employed by teams and leagues themselves. Such customs further entangle health care professionals in deep relationships with coaches and league officials, thereby intensifying the effects of motivated bias and COIs. These effects are not speculative; chapter 4 documents the lengthy history of the ways in which COIs and motivated bias have operated to the significant detriment of even professional (adult) tackle football players—let alone vulnerable youths and adolescents.

Because of the need to reimburse health care professionals for the services they render to tackle football participants, there is no way to entirely sequester health care professionals from all exchange and relationships with the American tackle football industry. Nevertheless, sequestration should be the guiding principle, and third-party payors should be used as much as possible to keep health care professionals at arms-length from the coaches, teams, and league officials whose priorities may not always be aligned with the best interests of the participants. At an absolute minimum, the practice by which health care professionals are directly sponsored, reimbursed, and even employed by teams and leagues must be rooted out and discontinued. It is embarrassing that the practice has persisted for so long in the face of its obvious and well-documented shortfalls.

Analysis of Policy Recommendation #3B

Although Policy Recommendation #3A is targeted at the health care professionals whose services are an absolute requirement for any adolescent participation in tackle football, the mandates for evidence-based COI policies should also apply to academic researchers and scientists. As both chapters 3 and 4 note, academics have long implicated themselves in the Manufacture of Doubt. Regulated industries implementing the script have sought partnerships with academic scientists and researchers primarily as a means of purchasing the credibility the industry lacks. Over the course of the twentieth century, this "doubt-making characteristic" (see chapter 3) has consistently proved successful in helping regulated industries achieve their political and economic objectives.

The justification for Policy Recommendation #3B follows both from this historical analysis and from the best evidence on motivated bias. Namely, it is simply not credible to claim that academics (or anyone else) can form deep relationships with a commercial industry and remain unlikely to exhibit behavior of partiality. Both experimental and natural evidence belie any such confidence in our ability to avoid behaving in ways that serve the interests of the parties with whom we are in deep relations. Moreover, the same bodies of evidence show that the only proven remedy for avoiding such behavior is to sequester the parties—to prevent the relationships that give rise to behaviors of partiality.[47]

Therefore, any academics who work in spaces that involve or implicate collision sports and the American tackle football industry in particular ought to implement a strategy of sequestration and eliminate relationships with that industry to the maximum extent possible. As is the case with Policy Recommendation #3A, sequestration is an orientation and a framing. There are contexts and situations where it may be impossible for academics to avoid all relationships with the tackle football industry. However, it should be noted that, unless they are health care professionals providing services to participants in tackle football, academics do not experience the same basic COI that arises from the need to reimburse health care professionals for the provision of health care services. For academics who are not service providers, there are many other situations in which relationships with regulated industries can arise, such as research funding.

To state an implication of Policy Recommendation #3A plainly: academics and university professors whose work centers on public and population health ought not accept research funding from regulated industries whose products are injurious to public health. The evidence driving this point is not dependent on any issue of optics, although, for example, concerns about how it "looks" for academics to be accepting money from tobacco companies to conduct research on lung cancer are certainly relevant. Rather, the justification for the claim that academics entering into relationships with the tackle football industry is ethically unacceptable flows from the two evidence bases mentioned above (the empirical evidence on motivated bias and COIs and the historicolegal evidence regarding the Manufacture of Doubt).

Because relationships with regulated industries motivate academics to be biased in favor of the interests and priorities of those industries, these relationships should be avoided wherever and whenever possible. Moreover, sponsored research and/or other forms of collaboration with regulated industries are a tried-and-true technique in the Manufacture of Doubt. Given this historical fact, academics who willingly enter into relationship with regulated industries can at a minimum fairly be charged with making it easier for regulated industries to manufacture doubt.

This is a critical point. Namely, even if we assume for argument's sake that academics and university-based researchers can enter into relationship with regulated industries without substantial risk of motivated bias and behavior of partiality, it would nevertheless be true that such acts perpetuate the Manufacture of Doubt.[48] The Manufacture of Doubt is a script, a kind of structural social phenomenon that is not reducible to the individual intentions of the actors participating in it. Regardless of the extent to which an academic or university-based researcher intends good faith, forming a relationship with a regulated industry literally constitutes an enactment of the social script that will often be of service for constructing ignorance. Indeed, the very formation of the relationship itself helps regulated industries manufacture doubt because doing so purchases social credibility for the industries (see chapter 3). Pharmaceutical companies prize the existence of relationships with prescribing physicians not only because of the outcome of a greater volume of prescriptions, but also because the mere fact of the relationship with respected academic physicians arrogates some of the immense credibility the latter enjoy to the pharmaceutical companies (that operate with significant credibility deficits).

The same phenomenon is true for virtually any regulated industry implementing the Manufacture of Doubt. Even if motivated bias was somehow unproblematic, the very fact of forming a relationship with regulated industries lends credibility to such industries selling products that are adverse to population health. This fact alone licenses the ethical claim embodied in Policy Recommendation #3B. Academics and university-based researchers should not be in the business of donating credibility to regulated industries whose products cause health problems. Trust and trustworthiness are important virtues that can only be earned through practice. Actors, including industries, that are deemed untrustworthy based on patterns and practices that earn mistrust ought not be enabled to cosplay trustworthiness by sponsoring academics and university-based researchers. And academics and university-based researchers have an ethical obligation to prevent this extension of unearned credibility, especially when doing so furthers the Manufacture of Doubt.

It is these kinds of considerations that have increasingly led public health organizations to reject the formation of relationships with regulated industries such as tobacco and alcohol. In response to the 2017 formation of the Foundation for a Smoke-free World, funded almost entirely by tobacco company Philip Morris International, the World Health Organization (WHO) reiterated that it would not partner with any health foundation funded by the tobacco industry.[49] The statement reminded readers that implementation guidelines for Article 5.3 of the WHO Framework Convention on Tobacco Control "state clearly that governments should limit interactions with the tobacco industry and avoid partnership."[50] This guideline itself embodies a commitment to sequestration, and the same is true regarding academics and university-based researchers.

Furthermore, there are important distinctions between the COIs experienced by individual academics and researchers and those experienced by institutions. In 2008, the *New York Times* reported on a problematic contract signed by Virginia Commonwealth University (VCU) with Philip Morris International. The contract governed an agreement to conduct research, and it contained data secrecy and industry control provisions that unquestionably violated university policy and consensus ethical standards. Specifically, the contract "bar[red] professors from publishing the results of their studies, or even talking about them, without Philip Morris's permission."[51] It also allocated virtually all of the patents and intellectual property rights to the tobacco company. When pressed for an explanation as to how the university could enter into a contract that its own policies specifically forbade for its faculty and researchers, the university demurred, stating that "in the end, it was language we thought we could agree to. It's a balancing act."[52]

The better explanation for VCU's conduct is that the university, which has existed as a medical college since 1838, is based in Richmond and has had a long and deep relationship with the (also) Richmond-based Philip Morris International. The depth and power of this relationship are the antecedent acts that created favorable dispositions towards the tobacco company, and that, as revealed in the 2008 *New York Times* investigation, resulted in behavior of partiality in favor of the tobacco company's commercial interests. The COIs present in this case study did not bias any individual faculty or investigator; they existed at the institutional level between the university itself and the regulated industry.

Recognizing that the same kinds of relationships can motivate institutions at the highest levels to biased behavior in favor of commercial industries suggests that Policy Recommendation #3B should not merely govern relationships between individual academics or university-based researchers but also centers, institutes, and public-private partnerships to which institutions of higher education are parties. Sequestration should be a guiding principle for ethical governance of all these possible relationships; wherever possible, such relationships should be prevented or eliminated entirely. Failing these ethically preferable choices, such relationships should be minimized to the maximum extent possible (which requires sequestering the parties and limiting the depth and extent of their entanglement as much as possible).

Policy Recommendation #4: Untether Tackle Football from Primary and Secondary Schools

No primary or secondary public schools shall sponsor a tackle football team.

In a 2016 feature titled "Friday Night Lights Out," journalist Patrick Hruby wondered why primary and secondary public schools in the US commonly sponsor tackle football teams. Note that this is a separate issue from parents choosing to enroll their children in private, tackle football leagues, or at least leagues not associated with a school. Such private enrollment is itself beset with ethical concerns that comprise the bulk of this book. Yet, encouraging schools to field tackle football teams is in essence "ask[ing] schools to sponsor a concussion delivery system, and . . . ask[ing] taxpayers to pick up the tab."[53] While neither boxing nor mixed martial arts in the US are considered deep play, if schools were to sponsor these types of activities that exposed participants to such obvious health harms, presumably at least some parents and families would be concerned. Why should tackle football be regarded any differently? Its status as deep play may explain, but can hardly justify, a widely divergent policy approach to preventing and managing the health harms associated with participating in the activity.

In a 2018 essay, ethicists Randall Curren and J. C. Blokhuis (who is also a legal scholar) lay out a detailed argument for why public schools have absolutely no moral justification for sponsoring American tackle football. They begin by noting that some aspects of the cultural resonance of deep play (which have helped solidify football's status as deep play) are incompatible with the goals of juvenile education:

Football players are indoctrinated into an oppressive system of norms that is hard to reconcile with the purposes of educational institutions. Players are schooled in conformity and notions of courage, glory, self-sacrifice, and stoic endurance of pain—notions, not virtues, because the sacrifice of young bodies and minds is not remotely justified by the glory of winning a game or the objective merits of well-executed plays and "wicked hits."[54]

In late November 2021, the *Orange County Register* ran a disturbing story from Santa Ana, California, about the high school football program at Mater Dei High School, "the largest coeducational Roman Catholic school west of the Mississippi River."[55] At the time of the story, Mater Dei's tackle football program ranked number one in the US by media outlets. In February 2021, the Santa Ana Police Department had contacted the school and requested information about an incident that had left an unnamed player (referred to for privacy purposes only as "Player #1") with "a traumatic brain injury, two gashes over his right eye, one over his left, and a broken nose that would require surgery."[56]

Since February, Player #1 had continued to experience problems related to his TBI and eventually withdrew from the school. Nevertheless, Mater Dei High School did not respond to the Santa Ana Police Department's request for information until April 2021. In November 2021, the family of Player #1 filed a lawsuit against both Mater Dei High School and the Roman Catholic Diocese of Orange. According to the news story, neither the head coach nor any other team or school officials undertook any response to the incident; indeed, the suit alleges, the injuries arose out of a hazing tradition on the team called "Bodies" or "Slappies" in which two players face each other and repeatedly punch each other in the torso.[57]

Worse yet, the suit further alleges that the Mater Dei athletic trainer did not immediately come to Player #1's aid even after witnessing the severity of his injuries, and instead "continued taping other players' ankles for practice."[58] Allegedly, the athletic trainer was further instructed by the administrative staff at the school "not to call the paramedics and to delay contacting (Player #1's) parents."[59] Mater Dei commissioned an independent probe of its athletics program but announced in January

2023 that it would not publicly release the summary report, just as it was finalizing a settlement of Player #1's lawsuit.[60] The *Orange County Register* article of January 2023 also dryly observed that "Mater Dei is currently named in at least nine ongoing lawsuits alleging sexual abuse by school employees."[61]

Although Player #1's injuries and withdrawal from the school are fact, the confidential nature of the settlement precludes public evaluation of the truth of the remainder of these allegations. Yet, if true, they reveal all too much. First, there is the shockingly familiar behavioral pattern by which adults charged with the health, safety, and well-being of their players prioritize other interests. For example, the 2021 *Register* news story reports that the father of Player #1 was told directly by the head coach that the coach was unable to take disciplinary action against Player #2 because Player #2's father was a voluntary coach with the team.[62]

Second, these events show the predictable and repeated evidence of behavior of partiality flowing from the COIs and motivated bias that have consistently—with literally brutal effectiveness—resulted in the very people most responsible for the health and safety of the players abandoning such responsibilities. Such behavior of partiality is perhaps most disturbing in the conduct of health care professionals who assume under both ethics and law additional fiduciary duties of care to place the best interests of their patients above all other competing interests. Unfortunately, the history of health professional response and management to tackle football injuries shows beyond question that these failures are common. In turn, the commonality of these failures reveals the existence of structural forces (here, the relationships with team and school officials) that explain why so many health care professionals have not met their fiduciary responsibilities. It is the existence of these forces, and the difficulty of rooting them out, that justify Policy Recommendation #3A which would disentangle and separate health care professionals from direct supervision or reimbursement from the teams, programs, leagues, and officials that sponsor play.

Third, the allegations in the *Register* account of the Mater Dei football program also highlight some key deficiencies in the tendency to highlight the social and cultural benefits of participation in collision sports and/or tackle football in particular. To be clear, youth and adolescent participation in team sports can and does bring a variety of benefits to individual participants, families, and communities. But while participation can promote virtues like teamwork and stress relief, the cultures that make tackle football deep play also often nurture a host of vices such as violence, intimidation, and abuse. Curren and Blokhuis argue that "the emphasis on obedience and conformity in football is not favorable to the development of [good] judgment."[63] Although this is contestable, there are certainly no shortage of examples from which to conclude that such emphasis is both (1) common in American tackle football, and (2) poses serious risks to the safety and well-being of participants. Ultimately, it is inappropriate to discuss the social and cultural benefits of youth and adolescent participation in tackle football without including full and frank discussion of the distinct and well-documented tendency of tackle football culture to inculcate vicious behaviors.

Fourth, even if none of the above were true as to the cultures of tackle football in the US, the question remains why schools should nevertheless sponsor "concussion delivery systems" for youths and adolescents.[64] Curren and Blokhuis lay out a detailed argument that such sponsorship is unethical. They contend that it violates a "cognitive harm" principle: "Schools should not sponsor activities that are known to cognitively impair a significant percentage of students who participate in these activities."[65]

There are several factual premises contained in this proposition that proponents of school sponsorship of American tackle football might contest. For example, to what extent is it "known" that tackle football cognitively impairs a "significant" percentage of students? And what percentage of students is fairly deemed "a significant percentage"? Therefore, we can easily adjust this cognitive harm principle to minimize such objections: "Schools should not sponsor activities that substantially elevate the risks of cognitive impairment and inflammatory disease for a significant percentage of students who participate in these activities."

This book has argued repeatedly that the evidence regarding causal inference is more than sufficient to justify public health interventions via laws and policies such as Policy Recommendations #1–#3 here. But even if we "reduce" the empirical premise in the Curren and Blokhuis's cognitive harm principle to one of association, the strength of the correlative evidence is also more than sufficient to warrant the same levels of intervention (see chapter 5). The ultimate moral question is: What business do public schools have in sponsoring activities that expose participants to serious risks of long-term injury?

One response to this question is to assert the benefits of participation. But there is no evidence whatsoever that the benefits available from participation in team sports are specific to tackle football and cannot be accrued via participation in sports and activities that pose far lower risks of serious injury and harm. As noted above, the tendency among proponents of youth tackle football to emphasize the benefits of play is peculiar because it (1) ignores or downplays the harms and risks of play, and (2) consistently fails to grapple with the obvious fact that such benefits are simply not specific to tackle football. Curren and Blokhuis point out:

> Participation in sports can be a vehicle for learning self-discipline, diligence, teamwork, and other enabling or "performance" virtues (just as participation in musical ensembles can be). However, this would be an argument for enabling all children to participate in sports that do not cause them countervailing harm. . . . Surely any benefits associated with football could be equally well or better achieved through other activities such as music, dance, debate, public service, and pre-professional clubs.[66]

Moreover, Curren and Blokhuis explain that under traditional Anglo-American common law tradition, parents cannot "give consent that would morally or legally void the responsibilities of schools and public authorities to protect children's interests. . . . [S]chools cannot ethically put children's welfare at risk even if their parents consent."[67] This is critical since it establishes that schools owe their students moral duties, the sources for which are independent of the moral duties parents owe their children. Thus, even if we were to assume that the primary arguments in this book are mistaken and that parental autonomy to expose their children to elevated risks of harm outweighs our obligations to protect youths and adolescents from preventable harm, that claim does not confer any license upon schools to abandon their own, additional duties to protect children from harms within a school-based context.

It is ethically permissible to restrict parental autonomy in the case of participation of youth and adolescent tackle football by means of a public health law banning tackling for youths under the age of 14 (Policy Recommendation #1). But even if it were not so permissible, and parents had full moral authority to elect to expose their children to the risks of American tackle football, it does not follow that schools can essentially free-ride on that consent without moral or legal consequence. Schools have additional moral and legal obligations to protect the children who are required to attend; these obligations do not derive from parental rights and responsibilities, but are rooted in the general *parens patriae* responsibility that US states have to protect "the independent welfare and developmental requirements of every child."[68]

Finally, school sponsorship of American tackle football raises stark social justice issues. Recall that under Powers and Faden's health sufficiency model, factors that intensify densely-woven patterns of disadvantage are priorities for public health remediation. This book has already noted that the tendency of participation in tackle football to worsen existing racial inequalities in both TBI and inflammatory disease violates this criterion of social justice. Scholars have long noted the ways in which schools in the US widen already existing racial inequalities through the connection between schooling, discipline, and the carceral state (often referred to as "the school-to-prison pipeline").[69] It would be even more transgressive if sponsorship of tackle football teams were yet another mechanism by which racial health inequalities are deepened across the

US. Some argue that to deprive the least well-off from the opportunities tackle football affords is itself an injustice. But as Curren and Blokhuis point out, this argument is akin to "locating hazardous waste incinerators in blighted neighborhoods and counting voluntary acceptance of jobs at them as consent by workers to endure the effects of chronic toxic exposure. In both cases, the choices are compelled to the extent that an unjust distribution of opportunities deprives those who must subject themselves to harm of the better options available in a more just system."[70]

In short, the widespread sponsorship of American tackle football teams in primary and secondary schools across the US is ethically unacceptable. The traditions supporting such sponsorship are deeply rooted in US culture and society—high schools have become virtual "feeders" for college football programs, and high school football recruiting is a multimillion-dollar industry in its own right. This presents tremendous practical problems in untethering tackle football from schools, but such practical issues are not themselves ethical arguments supporting the status quo. Arguing as such is an obvious instance of the "is-ought" fallacy by which a current state of affairs is taken to stand in for the way the world ought to be. School sponsorship of American tackle football teams violates basic mandates of social justice and is unethical. If youth and adolescent participation in American tackle football is to continue at all, it ought not be sponsored by the public fisc and sanctioned by public schools.

×××

Building on chapters 1–5, chapter 6 offers four core policy recommendations rooted in public health law and a rigorous model of social justice. There is every reason to believe that, if implemented, this set of recommendations would have substantial health impact in reducing the deleterious effects of youth and adolescent participation in American tackle football. That said, such a prediction must be evaluated. Fortunately, there are a variety of tools available for measuring the health impact of changes in laws and policies. Political scientists and economists have pioneered many of these methods, but the emerging field of legal epidemiology also offers diverse methods and tools for assessing the efficacy of public health law interventions.

There are multiple lines of evidence discussed in this book that justify a strong belief and prediction that implementing these policies would reduce the adverse health impact of youth and adolescent participation in American tackle football. It is beyond dispute that law is a powerful social determinant of health. But the proof is in the pudding, and if rigorous evaluation does not bear this prediction out, then these interventions should be revisited, revised, and reformed as needed.

The final portion of this final chapter moves on to consider some likely objections to this suite of policy recommendations.

Objection #1: The Policy Recommendations Infringe on Parental Autonomy

The central and most obvious objection to the policy recommendations of the previous section is that they infringe on parental autonomy. As noted throughout this book, both social and legal norms in the US afford parents considerable latitude in the risks to which they are permitted to expose their children. The objections to a policy recommendation to ban tackling for children under the age of 14 therefore tend to trade on these traditions of parental autonomy.

Wherever states have drafted bills proposing such a policy, the strident opposition has consistently centered on the rights of parents to make decisions that expose their children to risks of harm. For example, in response to Connecticut's 2019 efforts to prohibit tackle football through seventh grade, opponents argued that weighing the risks and deciding whether children may be exposed to them was a decision for parents rather than politicians.[71] Opposition to a 2019 New York state bill tracked similar points: "This is a parent's choice."[72]

The principal response to this objection is to point out that it is completely circular. It simply asserts as a conclusion the critical point under debate. While it is a fact that the scope of parental autonomy in the US is wide, it is equally factual that there are limits to this interest. Indeed, the question of where these limits should be drawn regarding youth and adolescent participation in American tackle football has been the subject of this entire book. At what point do the health risks of such participation warrant public health legal and policy intervention that circumscribes parental autonomy?

This book has presented a series of arguments justifying the conclusion that parental autonomy cannot justify exposing youths and adolescents to the health risks that attend playing American tackle football. A response that asserts the primacy of parental autonomy is nothing more than a restatement of the problem! As such, the claim "parental autonomy is paramount" is not only a poor argument when offered in response to a series of justified claims for curbing such autonomy in a given case. Rather, the claim is literally no argument at all, but merely the assertion of a preferred conclusion. An argument consists of three components: (1) premises, (2) chains of inference, and (3) a conclusion. A conclusion standing alone is not an argument. But this is exactly what the response "parental autonomy is paramount" consists of.

Why does the scope of parental autonomy to expose children to health harms permit the serious risks associated with participation in collision sports in general and with American tackle football in particular? And again, a principal argument of this book is that the evidence of exposure-harm is more than sufficient to warrant public health action specifically in the form of law and policy interventions that will shelter children. An argument in rebuttal would either need to show why the factual premises supporting the arguments in this book are unsound or inapplicable, and/or why the factual premises somehow fail to compel the conclusion that parental autonomy ought to be curbed in this case. An argument in rebuttal would need to demonstrate why the values and interests embodied in the sphere of parental autonomy outweigh the powerful social justice claims militating in favor of curbing parental autonomy of exposing children and adolescents to the hazards that attend American tackle football.

A naked assertion that "parental autonomy is paramount" delivers none of these requirements. No premises are offered that drive a specific conclusion that the good of parental autonomy outweighs the harms that flow from encouraging youths and adolescents to repeatedly ram into each other as fast as possible for our entertainment. Instead, the notion of "parental autonomy" is uttered almost as an incantation that amplifies the social magic of deep play. While this process is fascinating and noteworthy from a sociological perspective, it is no ethical justification at all for the conclusion that parents should be permitted to expose their children to the health harms of American tackle football.

There may yet be a compelling and detailed justification for how and why the scope of parental autonomy should encompass a decision on whether youths and adolescents should play American tackle football. But that justification must be made rather than have its conclusion assumed, and the response typically offered by proponents of such play does not qualify as such a justification. Therefore, the objection fails.

Objection #2: Communities of Color May Endorse Youth and Adolescent Participation in American Tackle Football

Part of the justification for banning tackling for participants under the age of 14 (Policy Recommendation #1) is that youth and adolescent participation in American tackle football may expand racial health inequalities in the US (thereby violating social justice). It is of course true that American tackle football plays an important social role within many communities of color in the US. And, in fact, there is at least anecdotal evidence that some such communities have led opposition to legislative efforts to ban American tackle football for players under the age of 14. In 2022, Medicaid and poverty scholar Jamila Michener released the Racial Equity and Policy (REAP) Framework for assessing health policy.[73] In it, she warned against a facile conclusion that because

a given health policy disproportionately impacts people of color, it is necessarily racist and unjust: "The temptation may be toward simplicity, to
look at the effects of policy and designate a policy as racist if it disproportionately affects people of color negatively. This is certainly one important metric by which we can evaluate a policy's racial inequity (hence
the relevance of disproportionality), but it is not the only standard."[74]

It is possible to argue that the benefits communities of color derive
from the deep play status of American tackle football outweigh the
harms flowing from its potentially chronic and lifelong adverse health
impact. Michener points out that while disproportionality is one metric
for evaluating the racial impact of health policy choices, what she terms
"voice" is another.[75] Thus, where the voices of communities of color
adopt a certain risk calculus that supports the disproportionate adverse
health impact of youth and adolescent participation in American tackle
football, it is at least theoretically possible for such an adoption to satisfy standards of social justice.

While this analysis merits serious consideration, it is also highly
speculative. There is little good evidence that communities of color overall endorse youth and adolescent participation in full-contact collision
sports even given awareness of the disproportionate adverse health impact. At best, this objection supports the ethical imperative of voice and
representation in policymaking processes regarding collision sports and
American tackle football. Where people of color bear disproportionate
burdens of the adverse health impact of youth and adolescent participation in collision sports, ethical policymaking demands that their voices
are prioritized in the policymaking process.

It remains the case that participation in an activity that almost certainly will expand racial inequalities in neurological and rheumatologi-
cal health across the life span is ethically suspect under the social justice
analysis articulated in this chapter. As with any other ethical determination, this perspective is subject to qualification and revision—which
is a strength of sensitive and careful policy analysis rather than a weakness. But the ethical imperative of voice and representation does not by

itself license the inference that an activity that both diminishes overall population health and expands racial health inequalities is morally acceptable. Therefore, this objection fails.

Objection #3: A Lack of Sufficient Health Care Professionals May Increase Inequalities in Participation

As noted in the analysis above, Policy Recommendation #2 provides that inadequate access to a minimally sufficient level of health care services should be a bar to youth and adolescent participation in American tackle football. There are two possible objections to this recommendation.

First, the American tackle football industry is not responsible for structural deficiencies in health care professionals and/or health care access. Of course, at the highest levels there is no excuse or justification for well-resourced tackle football organizations, such as the NFL or universities sponsoring tackle football teams, for failing to provide minimally sufficient health care services. But the same cannot be said for less well-off leagues and communities who already struggle with insufficiencies in access to health care professionals and services.

Many of the ethical problems noted in this book are indeed caused by or at least actively perpetuated by the tackle football industry. The industry bears moral and, in some cases, legal responsibility for the harms it knowingly causes and/or perpetuates. But since tackle football leagues and teams bear no significant portion of the responsibility for causing structural deficiencies in the health care workforce, why should they be penalized severely for such shortages?

Second, prohibiting tackle football in the absence of minimally sufficient access to health care services risks expanding socioeconomic inequalities in sports participation itself. Granting that such participation confers social benefit, expanding inequalities in a social good therein violates the second prong of a twin aims social justice model. This argument raises an important point: any nonideal theory of social justice inevitably requires weighing competing social goods and harms. Under the health sufficiency model, ethically optimal public health policies are those that maximize the twin aims at the same time. But it does not follow that a policy intervention that maximizes only one is always unjust. There are many grades between ethically optimal and unjust. Thus, for example, we might affirm a law or policy that produces enormous population health benefits for everyone, but that also expands inequalities by only a relatively small amount.[76] Conversely, we might consider investing in a law or policy intervention that delivers significant health benefit only for a historically oppressed subgroup but accomplishes little to advance overall population health. (This would have the effect of compressing health inequities, so maximizing the second aim of the model but not the first.)

The key point, then, is that while an expansion of socioeconomic inequalities is sufficient to negate a claim that a particular law and policy intervention is ethically optimal, such does not automatically mean that the intervention is ethically unacceptable. Interventions that confer large overall health benefits while only marginally increasing inequalities might well be ethically desirable in a given context. That this kind of weighing is highly fact- and context- dependent follows from the need to move and act in the nonideal world.

Thus, while the possibility that proscribing American tackle football could expand socioeconomic inequalities in participation is important, it is not the end of the ethical inquiry. It must be weighed against the social goods intended and likely to result from enacting the policy. The availability of health care services is essential for the safety and well-being of youths and adolescents participating in collision sports.

Accordingly, the availability of minimally sufficient health care services and professionals produces significant health benefits and avoids both minor and potentially catastrophic health harms. This overwhelmingly favorable benefit-harm ratio for a vulnerable population (youths and adolescents, especially in resource-poor settings) outweighs the potential increase in socioeconomic inequalities in participation. The magnitude of the overall benefits for the very group put at risk by participation is simply staggering. Moreover, the weighing exercise here is also affected by the fact that the two kinds of benefits being weighed are not apposite. One side of the scale is assessing health benefits and harms while the other is evaluating the benefits of participation in sport. While both of these are social goods, the latter is fungible in a way that the former is not. Namely, it is possible to gain at least some of the benefits of sport participation without incurring the substantial risks of serious and long-term harm that attend participation in American tackle football and/or other collision sports without access to minimally sufficient health care services. In contrast, there is little way to alleviate the serious risks of playing collision sports, such as American tackle football, without access to minimally sufficient health care services.

Ultimately, while it is certainly not ideal to adopt policy interventions that might expand socioeconomic inequalities in sport, prohibiting participation in American tackle football absent access to minimally sufficient health care services is ethically mandatory. The significantly elevated risks of serious, potentially catastrophic harm to youths and adolescents under such conditions outweigh all other considerations. If teams and leagues are unable to guarantee for participants access to minimally sufficient health care services, youths and adolescents should be prohibited from playing American tackle football.

Objection #4: American Tackle Football Should Be Completely Banned for Youths and Adolescents

This objection comes from the other direction, arguing that, rather than the proposed policy recommendations being too stringent, they do not go far enough. Specifically, given the evidence surveyed in this book and the ample justification for public health intervention to curb the harms to youths and adolescents for participation, why not simply ban the risky activity outright? None of the policy recommendations in this chapter endorse such a ban, which means that, to some extent and in at least some capacity, this book suggests that it is ethically appropriate for youths and adolescents to play American tackle football. Perhaps, the objection goes, the evidence and arguments in the book are sufficient to justify an outright ban on an activity that impermissibly exposes vulnerable communities to serious risks of long-term harm. If so, the failure to endorse such a ban is problematic.

This objection is plausible, but it assumes a critical premise that ultimately derails the argument. Namely, it presumes that the policy recommendations suborn youths and adolescents under the age of 14 to play tackle football. Recall that Policy Recommendation #1 prohibits tackling among youths and adolescents under the age of 14. But the recommendation allows tackle football for participants between the ages of 15 and 18.

Although there are many definitions of "collision sports," common among them is the specific mens rea or mental state: a sport that "permits deliberate collision between players."[77] Another definition regards collision sports as "those during which routine, purposeful, body-to-body collisions occur as a legal and expected part of the game."[78] Given that such intentional collisions will be prohibited by Policy Recommendation #1 for participants under the age of 14, the activity unquestionably associated with the most serious risks of long-term morbidity and mortality is eliminated. Indeed, given the favorable evidence associated with the elimination of bodychecking among youth and adolescent ice hockey players in Canada, one would be justified in predicting a similarly significant risk reduction in all manner of injury among American football players under the age of 14 subsequent to the elimination of tackling.

To briefly return to Learned Hand's negligence formula discussed in this chapter ($B < PL$): as the predicted probability and magnitude of the harm decreases (after the elimination of tackling for those under the age of 14), the justification for the most far-reaching intervention—prohibition of the activity itself—also diminishes. The burden of banning American football even without tackling for youths and adolescents might be substantial enough to outweigh the marginal health increase that would attend specifically "banning play" over "banning tackling."

This is especially likely among communities in which the deep play aspect of American football is deeply rooted. Ultimately, the successful implementation of Policy Recommendation #1 puts an attempt to completely ban American football for youths and adolescents on weaker epistemic and persuasive grounds.[79]

Objection #5: Difficulties in Implementing the Policy Recommendations Neuter Their Impact

The ways in which political interests become "represented" in law and policy is complex. Some policies that are widely favored do not become enshrined in law or are not even made a policy priority. Thus, the fact that no state in the US has yet enacted a law banning tackling for players under the age of 14 should not be taken as evidence that the law as of yet lacks sufficient political support. Recent public opinion data is scant, but a 2019 poll in Massachusetts found that 75% of the state's registered voters deemed American tackle football "unsafe" for children before high school, and a similar percentage professed willingness to support further regulation of youth football.[80]

Regardless of the relative support among voters for banning tackling for players under the age of 14, it seems fair to assume significant pushback at local, county, state, regional, and perhaps even national levels against a ban on tackling. The deep play resonance of American tackle football ensures that an effort to strip American football of the components that most surely embody violence will encounter swift resistance. Embedded in deep social structures of masculinity, power, and militarism, a challenge to the violence inherent in tackling is a challenge to all of these social framings and the political economies that grow from and envelop the sport. Thus, one could object that Policy Recommendation #1 is unlikely to be implemented in many communities around the US; in some parts of the US, enactment may be near impossible.

For different reasons, similar objections based on implausibility or implementation problems could be leveled against Policy Recommendations #2 and #3 at least. As to a prohibition on play absent access to minimally sufficient health care services (Policy Recommendation #2): communities in resource-poor settings may, because of structural deprivation, be less likely to give up socially meaningful activities even when they expose members of the community to elevated risks of harm. This finding, which is widely documented among marginalized and oppressed communities, is often referred to as the social patterning of health behavior.[81] There are many explanations for this phenomenon, some centering on the sense of hopelessness and ennui that often haunt communities with historical trauma.[82] Regardless, the point is that the evidence on the social patterning of behavior justifies a prediction that communities likely to lack access to minimally sufficient health care services might also be less likely to support proposals like Policy Recommendation #2, even if they understand perfectly well that this elevates the risk of serious injury for youths and adolescents participating in American tackle football in their own community.

As to Policy Recommendation #3, US society tolerates extensive COIs in all manner of social contexts, from permitting US legislators to own stock to permitting physicians to hold ownership interests in hospitals and clinics to which they refer patients. It seems plausible to suggest that a society which tolerates and even encourages such COIs might be unlikely to support policy interventions that seek to eliminate or minimize the relationships that drive motivated bias.

The basic response to all of these objections is to refer back to a concept known as the "ethics of health policy paradox": what we can do may not be what we ought to do, and what we ought to do may not be what we can accomplish.[83] As I have previously argued, permitting what we can do to define what we ought to do perpetuates the naturalistic or "is-ought" fallacy. If we permit the class of what we can do to exhaust the set of what we ought to do, we justify the indefinite extension of the status quo regardless of its immoralities. Although practical problems in implementing ethically justified public health interventions are legitimate concerns, they do not permit us to escape basic moral obligations to pursue ethically mandatory or ethically optimal public health policies.

In addition, there are multiple reasons to pursue policies that have seemingly little chance to be enacted in the short to intermediate term.

First, policies have signaling effects that are distinct from the specific outcomes of policies themselves. In context of health policy, the simple act of regulating youth and adolescent American tackle football sends a signal about the relative safety of the activity itself.[84] This effect can change behavior regardless of the extent to which the relevant policy is enforced. Similarly, the fact that a growing number of states have drafted bills that would enact Policy Recommendation #1 sends an important signal even where political obstacles exist that have currently prevented such bills from becoming law.

Second, and related, policy enactment in general is a complex process that may not be feasible in any given time and space. John Kingdon's influential policy streams model posits that three separate policy streams must converge for a policy window to open:

1. The problem stream (a situation in need of remediation must be identified)
2. The policy stream (a policy intervention must exist that can be applied to the problem)
3. The political stream (political events, changes, or moments create an opportunity to address the problem via policy)[85]

Where these streams do not converge, the policy window does not open, and it may not be possible at that time to enact or implement a given policy. One of the obvious implications of the policy streams model is that stakeholders pushing for a specific policy change must organize strategically and maintain maximum readiness to push through a policy window when and if it opens (and to anticipate such a window opening). Therefore, that a given policy intervention does not seem feasible now is a poor justification for abandoning advocacy and organizing efforts. The implication of the policy streams model here is that the infeasibility of any of the policy recommendations developed in this chapter is the beginning rather than the end of the efforts to be made in their respective advocacy.

Ultimately, Objection #5 is fair for as far as it goes, but it does not go all that far. That is, there are indeed serious practical problems to be overcome before any of the policy recommendations here may be enacted and implemented. The existence of these problems is not a license for rejecting the strong ethical case in favor of each of them. In addition, there are powerful reasons for acting on each of these policy recommendations even in communities and contexts in which their enactment at the current moment seems unlikely (i.e., such action may send important signals and may also facilitate policy action when a window opens). While the ethics of health policy paradox is a real problem in public health ethics, law, and policy, simply choosing to focus on what can be done is no resolution of the paradox at all. It is rather a surrender of the commitment to bring the world of what is closer to the world of what ought to be.

Conclusion

The most ardent fans and opponents of American tackle football can likely agree on at least one point: the sport is violent. What this violence entails for public health is a matter of great dispute, but the violence is unquestionably part of the attraction of deep play in general. This book has argued that the ongoing debates regarding the propriety of American tackle football and collision sports in general for youths and adolescents must be properly situated in historical context. This context emphasizes the ways in which regulated industries have continually manufactured doubt to create and sustain regulatory vacuums. The American tackle football industry has hewed closely to the script, with particular emphasis on the technique perfected by the tobacco industry: denying causation between the exposure and the harm.

The fact that collision sports in general and tackle football in particular involve ritualized forms of violence suggests an important link with larger histories of industrial and occupational health: structural violence.[1] Structural violence is a critical umbrella concept for explaining the pathways between patterns of domination, oppression, and subordination and health outcomes. These patterns are the primary causes of health and its distribution in the US and globally, meaning that contemporary health inequalities are best explained in terms of these configurations of structural and institutionalized violence. Unsurprisingly, then, collision sports reflect and to some extent fuel inequalities along all manner of important social strata. For example, that the majority of tackle football players in the US are Black means that the injuries associated with participation will almost enlarge existing racial health inequalities in TBI, pain, and inflammatory disease. As another example, Stephen T. Casper and Kelly O'Donnell recently connected the social toleration of head injuries from the violence of collision sports to a similar social allowance for head injuries experienced overwhelmingly by women because of intimate partner violence.[2]

Consider the enormous sums of money that American college football players earn for their universities, almost none of which, until very recently, was available to the actual players themselves. Unsurprisingly, many commentators have labeled major college football a plantation economy, with mostly Black players risking significant injury for mostly white athletic officials and university executives.[3] In almost every state, the highest paid public official is the tackle football or basketball coach, and 2023 statistics show that 86.8% of head coaches within NCAA Division I football are white.[4]

While racism and tackle football is the subject of its own voluminous literature, the point here is that debates over tackle football and TBI require analysis not merely of the violence on the field but also of the structural violence that shapes larger patterns of injury and health associated with the commerce of regulated industries. In turn, structural violence and the dramatic health inequalities for which it is responsible raise strong concerns of social justice. Any commitment to social and/or health justice requires attention to the twin aims—the improvement of overall population health and the compression of health inequalities. Because the epidemiologic evidence shows that youth and adolescent participation in American tackle football likely fails both of these aims, substantial changes via public health laws and policies are recommended.

First, tackling should be prohibited for players under the age of 14 in American football. Second, minimally sufficient health care services are a prerequisite for tackle football games in which youths and adolescents participate. Third, governing bodies should implement a policy of sequestration between health care professionals who care for injured players and team officials. Academics and university professors should also implement a policy of sequestration between themselves and the tackle football industry. Fourth, primary and secondary schools should not sponsor tackle football teams. Based on the epidemiologic evidence, there is every reason to believe that these policy recommendations, if implemented, will advance the overall health of the population most at-risk from the harms of tackle football, as well as compressing health inequalities in TBI, chronic pain, and inflammatory disease across the life span.

I am under no illusions as to the extreme political and practical difficulties in implementing almost any of these four recommendations. Chapter 6 discussed these obstacles at length and explained why, from a public and population health ethics standpoint, those obstacles are little argument against the effort to advance ethically justified law and policy recommendations. The power of utopian thinking lies not in any ignorance of practical difficulties but rather in envisioning what a more just world might look like. The task before us is precisely the effort to make our current world look more like that just world. Laws and policies, so often used to entrench injustice and oppression, remain powerful social determinants of health. That power ought to be harnessed in ways that advance justice and equity.

×××

In some ways, I grieve the loss of tackle football in my life. I do not hate the sport. Quite the contrary, I grew up with as much passion for the sport as anyone, and it meant so much to my immigrant family because it helped us feel American. And while I feel no less a US citizen because of its absence in my life, I mourn the connections it helped to forge within my family. No longer can I discuss the latest tackle football news with my brothers and my father. That immense and rich topic of conversation that connected us all is gone, and I feel its loss.

Nevertheless, one of the lessons of justice is that it requires ongoing sacrifice from the more privileged. Admittedly, individual consumption decisions have little impact on structural violence. The NFL is in no way affected by my individual decision not to consume its product. But to paraphrase Lindsay F. Wiley and Lawrence O. Gostin, governance is the name of the activity through which we come together collectively to solve problems that we cannot solve individually.[5] The population-level perspective adopted in this book emphasizes the role of collective action through law and policy change to ameliorate the harms caused and the inequalities perpetuated by youth and adolescent participation in collision sports and American tackle football.

Ultimately, the foundational ethical question is: What kind of people do we want to be?

Acknowledgments

Writing a monograph is an enormous lift and is impossible without the support and encouragement of many people and communities. I am indebted first to my mentor and advisor throughout law school and graduate school, William J. Winslade. His patience, support, and insight are reflected in all of my work, but especially on the subject of traumatic brain injury, which he made central to his scholarship.

This book is a product of the feedback and exchange of the wider scholarly community working on this subject. Many thanks go to Stephen Casper, Kathryn Henne, Mary McDonald, Daniel Morrison, Cathy van Ingen, and Matt Ventresca. Special thanks go out to Kathleen Bachynski, who has patiently collaborated with and educated me since she was a graduate student.

Developing the public health law framework for this book would have been impossible without the perspective of my colleagues in this small but mighty field, including Jalayne Arias, Micah Berman, Scott Burris, Doron Dorfman, Lance Gable, Nicole Huberfeld, Heather McCabe, Benjamin Mason Meier, Seema Mohapatra, Wendy Parmet, Alexandra Phelan, Ross Silverman, Michael Sinha, Matiangai Sirleaf, Rick Weinmeyer, and Ruqaiijah Yearby. Jason Smith is dear to me as a friend and a health law colleague, and I owe him much. I am especially indebted to Lindsay Wiley for her brilliance, kindness, and steadfast support over the last decade.

Colleagues at the Brody School of Medicine and the Honors College at East Carolina University further nurtured the ideas and perspectives detailed in this book. I extend my sincere thanks to Kenneth DeVille, Todd Savitt, Maria Clay, Hellen Ransom, Greg Hassler, Janet Malek Weinstein, and Clint Parker.

The University of Colorado is an especially friendly place in which to conduct research on sport and public health, and I am grateful for the assistance of a number of colleagues across the Anschutz Medical Campus. Shale Wong, Larry Green, Frank DeGruy, Ben Miller, Lina Brou, and Emma Gilchrist contributed a great deal to my policy education and training. This book reflects their kind and expert tutelage. From Sarah Hemeida, I learned patience and passion in policy translation and in advocacy.

At the Center for Bioethics and Humanities, thanks go to Jackie Glover, Eric Campbell, Matt DeCamp, Christine Baugh, David Weil, Meleah Himber, Lisa Culhane, and Laurie Munro. These colleagues provided support and good cheer in finishing a book during a raging pandemic. Danielle Chaet is a constant source of friendship and hope. I am so grateful for her help.

Special thanks go to Matt Wynia for supporting the project and helping create the professional space needed to complete it.

To Therese "Tess" Jones, there is little language I can use to express the depths of my appreciation. Working with her has been one of the joys of my professional life and this book reflects her kindness, support, and guidance.

Closer to home, I am immensely grateful to my family for their support and patience in listening to me discuss ideas and arguments for the book over the last five years. My daughter, Maya, is a light unto herself and I am so proud to know her. My life partner, Yuko, has unfailingly supported all my professional endeavors and is more responsible than she knows for this book's existence. My parents and siblings feature prominently in the personal history that led to this project, as the book details. I owe them much.

I am also grateful to the brilliant students in the Speech & Debate program at the Denver School of the Arts for their support and interest in the ideas at the core of this book.

They, along with all my students since I began teaching formally in 2009, are the catalyst for my work. I am only a scholar-teacher because my students are willing to learn with me. I am humbled by the opportunity to share this book with them and the wider world.

Notes

Introduction

1. Jane Perlez, "9,706 New Citizens Hear Bush," *New York Times*, September 18, 1984, https://www.nytimes.com/1984/09/18/us/9706-new-citizens-hear-bush.html.

2. Greg Garber, "Wandering through the Fog," ESPN, January 27, 2005, https://www.espn.com/nfl/news/story?id=1972288.

3. Specifically, in both 2022 and 2023, FIFA rejected a proposal to permit the introduction of temporary substitutes into play when a player experiences a concussion. See Paul MacInnes, "FA to Push FIFA Again for Temporary Concussion Substitute Trial," *Guardian*, February 8, 2023, https://www.theguardian.com/football/2023/feb/08/fa-to-push-fifa-again-for-temporary-concussion-substitute-trial.

4. Greg Price, "Massachusetts Lawmakers Introduce Bill to Ban Youth Football," Daily Caller, October 23, 2019, https://dailycaller.com/2019/10/23/mass-lawmakers-ban-youth-football/.

5. Steve Henson, "Newsom Blocks Proposed Ban on Youth Tackle Football: 'Parents Have the Freedom to Decide,'" *Los Angeles Times*, January 17, 2024, https://www.latimes.com/california/story/2024-01-17/gavin-newsom-veto-youth-tackle-football-ban-california-bill.

6. Jennifer A. Reich, *Calling the Shots: Why Parents Reject Vaccines* (New York: New York University Press, 2018).

7. Council on Sports Medicine and Fitness, "Trampoline Safety in Childhood and Adolescence," *Pediatrics* 130, no. 4 (2012): 774–779.

8. Stephen T. Casper, "Punch-Drunk Slugnuts: Violence and the Vernacular History of Disease," *Isis* 113, no. 2 (2022): 266–288.

9. Bennet I. Omalu, Steven T. DeKosky, Ryan L. Minster, M. Ilyas Kamboh, Ronald L. Hamilton, and Cyril H. Wecht, "Chronic Traumatic Encephalopathy in a National Football League Player," *Neurosurgery* 57, no. 1 (2005): 128–134.

10. Talmud, Pirke Avot 2:16, trans. Joshua Kulp, Sefaria, https://www.sefaria.org/Pirkei_Avot.2.16?lang=bi (accessed October 15, 2023).

Chapter 1. Public Health History and the Manufacture of Doubt

1. Clifford Geertz, "Deep Play: Notes on the Balinese Cockfight," *Daedalus* 101, no. 1 (1972): 1–37.

2. In disciplines from sociology to injury epidemiology, the preferred nomenclature for the dominant form of "football" in the US specifically is "American tackle football." There is a scholarly effort to replace the term "America" or "American" wherever possible with "US" and "USian," as the former reduces much of the landmass of the Western Hemisphere to the nation-state. While I am sympathetic to this recommendation, situating the book in the scholarship on tackle football in particular provides some reason for adopting the terminology favored in those fields. Thus this book will generally use the phrase "American tackle football."

3. Natalia Cecire, "League of Extraordinary Gentlemen," *New Inquiry*, January 31, 2014, https://thenewinquiry.com/league-of-extraordinary-gentlemen/. Cecire also points out the gendered nature of deep play: "Women and foreigners are functionally excluded from the Balinese cockfight. The parade of NFL officials, coaches, doctors, and spokespersons—all men (mostly white) but for one or two lawyers— show how they are functionally excluded from football's deep play, too." The gender and gendered structure of American tackle football is both a cause and an effect of its status as deep play, and therefore merits careful scrutiny in the pages to come.

4. Paul E. Farmer, Bruce Nizeye, Sara Stulac, and Salmaan Keshavjee, "Structural Violence and Clinical Medicine," *PLOS Medicine* 3, no. 10 (2006): e449.

5. P. R. Lockhart, "How Slavery Became America's First Big Business," *Vox*, August 16, 2019, https://www.vox.com/identities/2019/8/16/20806069/slavery -economy-capitalism-violence-cotton-edward-baptist.

6. Götz Aly, *Hitler's Beneficiaries: Plunder, Racial War, and the Nazi Welfare State* (New York: Henry Holt, 2008).

7. Nancy Leong, "Racial Capitalism," *Harvard Law Review* 126 (2013): 2151.

8. Whitney Pirtle, "Racial Capitalism: A Fundamental Cause of Novel Coronavirus (COVID-19) Pandemic Inequities in the United States," *Health Education and Behavior* 47, no. 4 (2020): 504–508.

9. Bruce G. Link and Jo C. Phelan, "Conceptualizing Stigma," *Annual Review of Sociology* 27, no. 1 (2001): 363–385.

10. John Nightingale, "On the Definition of 'Industry' and 'Market,'" *Journal of Industrial Economics* (1978): 31–40, p. 32, quoting P.W.S. Andrews, *Manufacturing Business* (London: MacMillan, 1949): 178.

11. Nightingale, "On the Definition of 'Industry' and 'Market,'" 32, quoting Andrews, *Manufacturing Business*, 178.

12. Joseph D. Kearney and Thomas W. Merrill, "The Great Transformation of Regulated Industries Law," *Columbia Law Review* 98, no. 6 (1998): 1327, quoting Richard J. Pierce Jr. and Ernest Gellhorn, *Regulated Industries in a Nutshell*, 3d ed. (St. Paul, MN: West Publishing, 1994): 1.

13. See Federal Food, Drug, and Cosmetic Act of 1938, 21 U.S.C. ch. 9 § 309 and

following; Susanne M. Klausen and Julie Parle, "'Are We Going to Stand By and Let These Children Come into the World?': The Impact of the 'Thalidomide Disaster' in South Africa, 1960–1977," *Journal of Southern African Studies* 41, no. 4 (2015): 735–752; Henning Sjöström and Robert Nilsson, *Thalidomide and the Power of the Drug Companies* (New York: Penguin, 1972).

14. Katie Thomas, "The Story of Thalidomide in the US, Told through Documents," *New York Times*, March 23, 2020, https://www.nytimes.com/2020/03/23/health/thalidomide-fda-documents.html.

15. Jonathan T. Macy, Kyle Kercher, Jesse A. Steinfeldt, and Keisuke Kawata, "Fewer US Adolescents Playing Football and Public Health: A Review of Measures to Improve Safety and an Analysis of Gaps in the Literature," *Public Health Reports* 136, no. 5 (2021): 562–574.

16. Shannon Nutt, Lachlan Gillies, Marnee J. McKay, and Kerry Peek, "Neck Strength and Concussion Prevalence in Football and Rugby Athletes," *Journal of Science and Medicine in Sport* 25, no. 8 (2022): 632–638; James T. Ekner, Youkeun K. Oh, Monica S. Joshi, James K. Richardson, and James A. Ashton-Miller, "Effect of Neck Muscle Strength and Anticipatory Cervical Muscle Activation on the Kinematic Response of the Head to Impulsive Loads," *American Journal of Sports Medicine* 42, no. 3 (2014): 566–576.

17. Courtney Rozen, "AI Leaders Are Calling for More Regulation of the Tech. Here's What That May Mean in the US," *Washington Post*, May 31, 2023, https://www.washingtonpost.com/business/2023/05/31/regulate-ai-here-s-what-that-might-mean-in-the-us/770b9208-ffd0-11ed-9eb0-6c94dcb16fcf_story.html.

18. Dennis A. Gioia and Peter P. Poole, "Scripts in Organizational Behavior," *Academy of Management Review* 9, no. 3 (1984): 449–459, quote on p. 450, emphasis in original.

19. Gioia and Poole, "Scripts in Organizational Behavior," 454.

20. Gioia and Poole, "Scripts in Organizational Behavior," 454; see also Michael J. Oldani, "Uncanny Scripts: Understanding Pharmaceutical Emplotment in the Aboriginal Context," *Transcultural Psychiatry* 46, no. 1 (2009): 131–156; Rosa R. Krausz, "Organizational Scripts," *Transactional Analysis Journal* 23, no. 2 (1993): 77–86; Robert G. Lord and Mary C. Kernan, "Scripts as Determinants of Purposeful Behavior in Organizations," *Academy of Management Review* 12, no. 2 (1987): 265–277.

21. See Joseph Dumit, *Picturing Personhood: Brain Scans and Biomedical Identity* (Princeton, NJ: Princeton University Press, 2004).

22. Joelle M. Abi-Rached and Nikolas Rose, "The Birth of the Neuromolecular Gaze," *History of the Human Sciences* 23, no. 1 (2010): 11–36.

23. Nikolas Rose and Joelle M. Abi-Rached, *Neuro: The New Brain Sciences and the Management of the Mind* (Princeton, NJ: Princeton University Press, 2013).

24. Robert R. Edwards, Can Ozan Tan, Inana Dairi, Alicia J. Whittington, Julius Dewayne Thomas, Claudia M. Campbell et al., "Race Differences in Pain and Pain-Related Risk Factors among Former Professional American-style Football Players," *Pain* 164, no. 10 (2023): 2370–2379; Joel T. Fuller, et al., "High Prevalence of Dysfunctional, Asymmetrical, and Painful Movement in Elite Junior Australian Football Players Assessed Using the Functional Movement Screen," *Journal of Science and Medicine in Sport* 20, no. 2 (2017): 134–138.

25. Benjamin J. Morasco, Susan Gritzner, Lynsey Lewis, Robert Oldham, Dennis C. Turk, and Steven K. Dobscha, "Systematic Review of Prevalence, Correlates, and Treatment Outcomes for Chronic Non-Cancer Pain in Patients with Comorbid Substance Use Disorder," *Pain* 152, no. 3 (2011): 488–497.

26. Sara Baghikar, Amanda Benitez, Patricia Fernandez Piñeros, Yue Gao, and Arshiya A. Baig, "Factors Impacting Adherence to Diabetes Medication among Urban, Low Income Mexican-Americans with Diabetes," *Journal of Immigrant and Minority Health* 21 (2019): 1334–1341.

27. Neal Halfon, Shirley A. Russ, and Edward L. Schor, "The Emergence of Life Course Intervention Research: Optimizing Health Development and Child Well-Being," *Pediatrics* 149, Supplement 5 (2022): e2021053509C; Paula Braveman and Colleen Barclay, "Health Disparities Beginning in Childhood: A Life-Course Perspective," *Pediatrics* 124, Supplement_3 (2009): S163–S175; Lori G. Irwin, Arjumand Siddiqi, and Clyde Hertzman, "Early Childhood Development: A Powerful Equalizer," Final Report for the World Health Commission on the Social Determinants of Health, 2007, https://apps.who.int/iris/bitstream/handle/10665/69729/a91213.pdf;sequence=1.

28. See Susan E. Bell, *DES Daughters, Embodied Knowledge, and the Transformation of Women's Health Politics in the Late Twentieth Century* (Philadelphia: Temple University Press, 2009).

29. Vincent J. Felitti, R. F. Anda, D. Nordenberg, D. F. Williamson, A. M. Spitz, V. Edwards, M. P. Koss et al., "Relationship of Childhood Abuse and Household Dysfunction to Many of the Leading Causes of Death in Adults: The Adverse Childhood Experiences (ACE) Study," *American Journal of Preventive Medicine* 14, no. 4 (1998): 245–258.

30. For example, childhood and school vaccine mandates have a long history in the US, extending back to the last quarter of the nineteenth century. Elena Conis, "The History of the Personal Belief Exemption," *Pediatrics* 145, no. 4 (2020): e20192551. In contrast, adult vaccine mandates remained relatively rare until the COVID-19 pandemic, and given their unpopularity and judicial skepticism of such mandates, they are likely to remain rare. See Wendy Parmet, *Constitutional Contagion: COVID, the Courts, and Public Health* (Cambridge: Cambridge University Press, 2023).

31. Nitin Agarwal, Rut Thakkar, and Khoi Than, eds., "Concussion," American

Association of Neurological Surgeons, https://www.aans.org/Patients/Neurosurgical
-Conditions-and-Treatments/Concussion (last accessed February 1, 2024).

32. Zack Furness, "Reframing Concussions, Masculinity, and NFL Mythology
in League of Denial," *Popular Communication* 14, no. 1 (2016): 49–57; Amanda Turk,
"'We Have Work to Do, and We're Doing It': An Analysis of Roger Goodell's Rhetoric
During the NFL's Ongoing Concussion Crisis" (PhD diss., University of Kansas, 2017);
Daniel Kenzie, "Defining Injury, Managing Uncertainty: Articulating Definitions of
Traumatic Brain Injury" (PhD diss., Purdue University, 2017); Josh Compton and
Jordan Compton, "Open Letters from the National Football League, Concussion
Prevention, and Image-Repair Rhetoric," *International Journal of Sport Communica-
tion* 8, no. 3 (2015): 266–275.

33. Kathleen E. Bachynski and Daniel S. Goldberg, "Youth Sports & Public
Health: Framing Risks of Mild Traumatic Brain Injury in American Football and
Ice Hockey," *Journal of Law, Medicine & Ethics* 42, no. 3 (2014): 323–333.

Chapter 2. The Manufacture of Doubt and Its Proponents

1. Silvia De Renzi, "Witnesses of the Body: Medico-Legal Cases in Seventeenth-
Century Rome," *Studies in History and Philosophy of Science Part A* 33, no. 2 (2002):
219–242.

2. Daniel S. Goldberg, "Doubt & Social Policy: The Long History of Malingering
in Modern Welfare States," *Journal of Law, Medicine & Ethics* 49, no. 3 (2021): 385–393.

3. Michel Foucault, *The Birth of the Clinic: An Archaeology of Medical Perception*,
trans. Alan Sheridan (New York: Vintage Books, 1994).

4. See Lorraine Daston and Peter Galison, *Objectivity* (New York: Zone Books,
2007).

5. Daniel S. Goldberg, "Suffering and Death among Early American Roentgenologists: The Power of Remotely Anatomizing the Living Body in Fin de siècle America," *Bulletin of the History of Medicine* 85, no. 1 (2011): 1–28.

6. Goldberg, "Suffering and Death"; see also Daniel Goldberg, "'What They
Think of the Causes of So Much Suffering': S. Weir Mitchell, John Kearsley Mitchell,
and Ideas about Phantom Limb Pain in Late 19th c. America," *Spontaneous Generations:
A Journal for the History and Philosophy of Science* 8, no. 1 (2016): 27–54; Daniel S.
Goldberg, "The Transformative Power of X-Rays in US Scientific & Medical Litigation: Mechanical Objectivity in *Smith v. Grant* (1896)" *Perspectives on Science* 21, no. 1
(2013): 23–57.

7. See Tanya Sheehan, *Doctored: The Medicine of Photography in Nineteenth-century
America* (Happy Valley: Pennsylvania State University Press, 2011).

8. Jennifer L. Mnookin, "The Image of Truth: Photographic Evidence and the
Power of Analogy," *Yale Journal of Law & the Humanities* 10 (1998): 1.

9. See Goldberg, "Doubt & Social Policy."

10. See Mark Aldrich, *Death Rode the Rails: American Railroad Accidents and Safety, 1828–1965* (Baltimore: Johns Hopkins University Press, 2006); Ralph Harrington, "The Railway Accident: Trains, Trauma and Technological Crisis in Nineteenth Century Britain," in *Traumatic Pasts: History, Psychiatry, and Trauma in the Modern Age, 1870–1930,* ed. Mark S. Micale and Paul Lerner (Cambridge: Cambridge University Press, 2001): 31–56; Eric Caplan, "Trains and Trauma in the American Gilded Age," in *Traumatic Pasts: History, Psychiatry, and Trauma in the Modern Age, 1870–1930,* ed. Mark S. Micale and Paul Lerner (Cambridge: Cambridge University Press, 2001): 57–80; Eric Michael Caplan, "Trains, Brains, and Sprains: Railway Spine and the Origins of Psychoneuroses," *Bulletin of the History of Medicine* 69, no. 3 (1995): 387–419.

11. Nate Holdren, *Injury Impoverished: Workplace Accidents, Capitalism, and Law in the Progressive Era* (Cambridge: Cambridge University Press, 2020): 51.

12. See Steven W. Usselman, *Regulating Railroad Innovation: Business, Technology, and Politics in America, 1840–1920* (Cambridge: Cambridge University Press, 2002); but see Herbert Hovenkamp, "Regulatory Conflict in the Gilded Age: Federalism and the Railroad Problem," *Yale Law Journal* 97, no. 6 (1987): 1017–1072 (arguing that a simplistic regulatory capture model fails to explain the complexity of railroad regulation in the Gilded Age).

13. Usselman, *Regulating Railroad Innovation.*

14. See Kenneth A. DeVille, *Medical Malpractice in Nineteenth-Century America: Origins and Legacy* (New York: New York University Press, 1992).

15. In terms of nineteenth-century US legal history, it is typically difficult to know the number of cases actually brought. Petitions or pleas (the documents that generally initiate tort litigation in Anglo-American common law) were only infrequently preserved and are generally not indexed in any centralized codex or database. Moreover, petitions or pleas tell us nothing about the disposition of a given case. Absent a judgment, appeal, and the rendering of an appellate decision, which creates a record that forms the basis of *stare decisis* in the US, it is often difficult to know many details about tort cases of the nineteenth century.

16. See Paul Starr, *The Social Transformation of American Medicine* (New York: Basic Books, 1982).

17. See Katherine Keisler-Starkey and Lisa N. Bunch, "Health Insurance Coverage in the United States: 2021," US Census Bureau, Report Number P60–278, September 13, 2022, https://www.census.gov/library/publications/2022/demo/p60-278.html.

18. See Herbert K. Abrams, "A Short History of Occupational Health," *Journal of Public Health Policy* 22, no. 1 (2001): 34–80.

19. Alison Bashford and Carolyn Strange, "Thinking Historically About Public Health," *Medical Humanities* 33, no. 2 (2007): 87–92.

20. Michael Crichton, *Timeline* (New York: Random House, 2013): 82.

21. Starr, *Social Transformation*, 200–204.

22. Aldrich, *Death Rode the Rails*, 167.

23. For extensive discussion of the professionalization of industrial physicians, see Holdren, *Injury Impoverished*, 222–227.

24. Holdren, *Injury Impoverished*, 218.

25. *Accident and Injury: Their Relations to Diseases of the Nervous System* (New York: D. Appleton & Company, 1898): 344.

26. *Spinal Concussion: Surgically Considered as a Cause of Spinal Injury, and Neurologically Restricted to a Certain Symptom Group, for Which Is Suggested the Designation, Erichsen's Disease, as one Form of Traumatic Neurosis* (Philadelphia: F. A. Davis, 1889): 271.

27. *Spinal Concussion*, 272.

28. *Injuries of the Spine and Spinal Cord without Apparent Mechanical Lesion, and Nervous Shock: In Their Surgical and Medico-Legal Aspects* (London: J. A. Churchill, 1883): 235.

29. See Ralph Harrington, "On the Tracks of Trauma: Railway Spine Reconsidered," *Social History of Medicine* 16, no. 2 (2003): 209–223.

30. Harrington, "On the Tracks of Trauma."

31. See Goldberg, "Doubt & Social Policy"; Daniel S. Goldberg, "Pain, Objectivity and History: Understanding Pain Stigma," *Medical Humanities* 43, no. 4 (2017): 238–243.

32. Harrington, "On the Tracks of Trauma."

33. Harrington, "On the Tracks of Trauma," 214.

34. See Goldberg, "Pain, Objectivity, and History"; Goldberg, "Suffering and Death among Early American Roentgenologists."

35. See Nikolas Rose and Joelle M. Abi-Rached, *Neuro: The New Brain Sciences and the Management of the Mind* (Princeton, NJ: Princeton University Press, 2013).

36. David P. McCabe and Alan D. Castel, "Seeing Is Believing: The Effect of Brain Images on Judgments of Scientific Reasoning," *Cognition* 107, no. 1 (2008): 343–352.

37. See Holdren, *Injury Impoverished*, 175–217.

38. Sir John Collie, *Malingering and Feigned Sickness* (London: Edward Arnold, 1913).

39. David Rosner and Gerald Markowitz, *Deadly Dust: Silicosis and the Politics of Occupational Disease in Twentieth-century America* (Princeton, NJ: Princeton University Press, 1994): 7.

40. Rosner and Markowitz, *Deadly Dust*, 31

41. Rosner and Markowitz, *Deadly Dust*, 31.
42. Rosner and Markowitz, *Deadly Dust*, 43.
43. Rosner and Markowitz, *Deadly Dust*, 66.
44. Rosner and Markowitz, *Deadly Dust*, 67.
45. Rosner and Markowitz, *Deadly Dust*, 67.
46. Rosner and Markowitz, *Deadly Dust*, 69.
47. Rosner and Markowitz, *Deadly Dust*, 69.
48. Rosner and Markowitz, *Deadly Dust*, 81.
49. Rosner and Markowitz, *Deadly Dust*, 84.
50. Rosner and Markowitz, *Deadly Dust*, 96.
51. Rosner and Markowitz, *Deadly Dust*, 103.
52. Daniel Carpenter and David A. Moss, eds., *Preventing Regulatory Capture: Special Interest Influence and How to Limit It* (Cambridge: Cambridge University Press, 2014): 1.
53. Mark Tushnet, "Introduction: The Pasts & Futures of the Administrative State," *Daedalus* 150, no. 3 (2021): 5–16.
54. See Theodore H. Cohn, "The Effects of Regulatory Capture on Banking Regulations: A Level-of-Analysis Approach," in *The Failure of Financial Regulation: Why a Major Crisis Could Happen Again*, ed. A. Hira, N. Gaillard, and T. Cohn (London: Palgrave Macmillan 2019): 71–110; Carpenter and Moss, *Preventing Regulatory Capture*; Jed Goodfellow, "Regulatory Capture and the Welfare of Farm Animals in Australia," *Animal Law and Welfare—International Perspectives* (2016): 195–235.
55. See Rosner and Markowitz, *Deadly Dust*, 110.
56. Rosner and Markowitz, *Deadly Dust*, 111.
57. Rosner and Markowitz, *Deadly Dust*, 129.
58. Rosner and Markowitz, *Deadly Dust*, 126.
59. Rosner and Markowitz, *Deadly Dust*, 126.
60. Jock McCulloch, "Sleights of Hand: South Africa's Gold Mines and Occupational Disease," *New Solutions: A Journal of Environmental and Occupational Health Policy* 25, no. 4 (2016): 469–479, quote on p. 473.
61. McCulloch, "Sleights of Hand," 474.
62. See Rosner and Markowitz, *Deadly Dust*, 133.
63. Rosner and Markowitz, *Deadly Dust*, 133.
64. Rosner and Markowitz, *Deadly Dust*, 179.
65. Rosner and Markowitz, *Deadly Dust*, 204.
66. See Robert Proctor, *Golden Holocaust: Origins of the Cigarette Catastrophe and the Case for Abolition* (Berkeley: University of California Press, 2012); Linsey McGoey, *The Unknowers: How Strategic Ignorance Rules the World* (London: Bloomsbury Publishing, 2019).

67. Proctor, *Golden Holocaust*, 289.

68. Proctor, *Golden Holocaust*, 290–292.

69. Allan Brandt, *The Cigarette Century: The Rise, Fall, and Deadly Persistence of the Product That Defined America* (New York: Basic Books, 2009): 160.

70. Brandt, *Cigarette Century*, 169.

71. Brandt, *Cigarette Century*, 170.

72. Brandt, *Cigarette Century*, 170.

73. Brandt, *Cigarette Century*, 170.

74. Brandt, *Cigarette Century*, 171.

75. One might contest the tightness of the idea of capture with legislators since they do not stand in the same relationship with the industry as regulators. Nevertheless, public interest theory makes plain the ways that sophisticated political (industrial) actors form relationships with members of the House of Representatives and the Senate in the hopes of influencing alliances, positions, and the legislative machinery itself.

76. Peter D. Jacobsen, Jeffrey Wasserman, and John R. Anderson, "Historical Overview of Tobacco Legislation and Regulation," *Journal of Social Issues* 53, no. 1 (1997): 75–95, quote on p. 76.

77. Jacobsen et al., "Historical Overview," 77.

78. Jacobsen et al., "Historical Overview," 81.

79. Proctor, *Golden Holocaust*, 357–389.

80. See Howard Koh and Michael Fiore, "The Tobacco Industry and Harm Reduction," *JAMA* 328, no. 20 (2022): 2009–2010. As Koh and Fiore note, this particular strategy seeks to co-opt harm reduction language and frameworks, essentially arguing that the industry's preferred outcome actually advances public and population health.

81. David Heath, "Contesting the Science of Smoking," *The Atlantic*, May 4, 2016, https://www.theatlantic.com/politics/archive/2016/05/low-tar-cigarettes/481116/.

82. David Nye, "Regulatory Myopia and Public Health: 'Tough' Tobacco Control?," *Competition & Change* 8, no. 3 (2004): 305–321, quote on p. 310.

83. FDA v. Brown & Williamson Tobacco Corp., 529 U.S. 120 (2000).

84. 21 U.S.C. § 387-a and following; Family Smoking Prevention and Tobacco Control Act of 2009, Pub. L. 111-31.

85. See Robert Proctor, "The History of the Discovery of the Cigarette–Lung Cancer Link: Evidentiary Traditions, Corporate Denial, Global Toll," *Tobacco Control* 21, no. 2 (2012): 87–91. Proctor, *Golden Holocaust*.

86. Proctor, "History of the Discovery," 89.

87. Proctor, "History of the Discovery," 89.

88. Proctor, "History of the Discovery," 89.

89. Yussuf Saloojee and Elif Dagli, "Tobacco Industry Tactics for Resisting Public Policy on Health," *Bulletin of the World Health Organization* 78 (2000): 902–910, quote on p. 903.

90. Sharon Milberger, Ronald M. Davis, Clifford E. Douglas, John K. Beasley, David Burns, Thomas Houston, and Donald Shopland, "Tobacco Manufacturers' Defence Against Plaintiffs' Claims of Cancer Causation: Throwing Mud at the Wall and Hoping Some of It Will Stick," *Tobacco Control* 15, no. suppl 4 (2006): iv17–iv26.

91. Milberger et al., "Tobacco Manufacturers' Defence," iv23.

92. Robert K. Jackler, "Testimony by Otolaryngologists in Defense of Tobacco Companies 2009–2014," *The Laryngoscope* 125, no. 12 (2015): 2722–2729, quote on pp. 2727–2728.

93. Milberger et al., "Tobacco Manufacturers' Defence," iv23.

94. Milberger et al., "Tobacco Manufacturers' Defence," iv23.

Chapter 3. The American Tackle Football Industry's Manufacture of Doubt

1. Adam M. Finkel, Chris Deubert, Orly Lobel, I. Glenn Cohen, and Holly Fernandez Lynch, "The NFL as a Workplace: The Prospect of Applying Occupational Health and Safety Law to Protect NFL Workers," *Arizona Law Review* 60 (2018): 291.

2. It is fair to note that this argument is a dependent claim. That is, it depends for its validity on the extent to which a key premise is sound: that the American tackle football industry practices the Manufacture of Doubt. If it does not, then one cannot reasonably claim the (nonexistent) use of the script is evidence of a regulated industry. The analysis has been demarcated into two separate questions primarily for ease of reference (whether American tackle football is a regulated industry, and if so, whether that industry manufactures doubt). Yet they are not conceptually distinct inquiries, so the dependence of this particular claim is not itself problematic for my argument. As this chapter shows, the American tackle football industry has unquestionably plied the Manufacture of Doubt. Therefore both of the dependent claims are valid.

3. Dennis Dodd, "College Football Takes Aim at Its Greatest Issues as It Tries to Reinvent the Game for the Future," CBS Sports (website), August 22, 2019, https://www.cbssports.com/college-football/news/college-football-takes-aim-at-its-greatest-issues-as-it-tries-to-reinvent-the-game-for-the-future/.

4. Daniel S. Goldberg, "Eschewing Definitions of the Therapeutic Misconception: A Family Resemblance Analysis," *Journal of Medicine and Philosophy* 36, no. 3 (2011): 296–320, quote on p. 301, emphasis added.

5. Goldberg, "Eschewing Definitions," 302.

6. Kathleen E. Bachynski and Daniel S. Goldberg, "Time out: NFL Conflicts of

Interest with Public Health Efforts to Prevent TBI," *Injury Prevention* 24, no. 3 (2018): 180–184; Daniel S. Goldberg, "Concussions, Professional Sports, and Conflicts of Interest: Why the National Football League's Current Policies are Bad for Its (Players') Health," *HEC Forum* 20 (2008): 337–355.

7. See Rebecca L. Haffajee, "The Public Health Value of Opioid Litigation," *Journal of Law, Medicine & Ethics* 48, no. 2 (2020): 279–292; Adam D. K. Abelkop, "Tort Law as an Environmental Policy Instrument," *Oregon Law Review* 92 (2013): 381; Thomas Koenig and Michael Rustad, *In Defense of Tort Law* (New York: New York University Press, 2001).

8. Christopher R. Deubert, I. Glenn Cohen, and Holly Fernandez Lynch, "Protecting and Promoting the Health of NFL Players: Legal and Ethical Analysis and Recommendation," *The Football Players Health Study at Harvard University*, November 2016, https://footballplayershealth.harvard.edu/law-and-ethics-protecting-and -promoting/executive-summary/.

9. See generally Daniel S. Goldberg, "Doubt & Social Policy: The Long History of Malingering in Modern Welfare States," *Journal of Law, Medicine & Ethics* 49, no. 3 (2021): 385–393.

10. Patrick Hruby, "The NFL Concussion Settlement Is Pure Evil," *VICE*, October 28, 2014, https://www.vice.com/en/article/aem94g/the-nfl-concussion-settlement-is -pure-evil.

11. Andrew Heisel, "That Time an NFL Team Used Truth Serum on an Injured Player," *VICE*, December 3, 2014, https://www.vice.com/en/article/xyj3yn/that-time -an-nfl-team-used-truth-serum-on-an-injured-player.

12. Heisel, "That Time an NFL Team Used Truth Serum."

13. Heisel, "That Time an NFL Team Used Truth Serum."

14. Derek Marks, "One for Twenty-Five: The Federal Courts Reverse a Decision of the NFL's Disability Board for the First Time Since 1993 in *Jani v. Bert Bell/Pete Rozelle NFL Player Retirement Plan*," *Villanova Sports & Entertainment Law Journal* 15 (2008): 1.

15. Cecil R. Reynolds and Arthur MacNeill Horton Jr., eds., *Detection of Malingering during Head Injury Litigation* (Springer, 2021).

16. Steve P. Calandrillo, "Sports Medicine Conflicts: Team Physicians vs. Athlete-Patients," *St. Louis University Law Journal* 50 (2005): 185–201, quote on p. 192.

17. *League of Denial: The N.F.L.'s Concussion Crisis*, directed by Michael Kirk, aired October 8, 2013, on PBS Frontline, https://www.youtube.com/watch?v=SedClkAnclk.

18. James Andrew Miller and Ken Belson, "N.F.L. Pressure Said to Lead ESPN to Quit Film Project," *New York Times*, August 23, 2013, https://www.nytimes.com/2013 /08/24/sports/football/nfl-pressure-said-to-prompt-espn-to-quit-film-project.html.

19. Miller and Belson, "N.F.L Pressure."

20. Miller and Belson, "N.F.L Pressure."

21. Miller and Belson, "N.F.L Pressure."

22. Mark Fainaru-Wada and Steve Fainaru, *League of Denial: The NFL, Concussions, and the Battle for Truth* (United States: Crown, 2014).

23. Peter Keating, "Doctor Yes," *ESPN The Magazine*, November 6, 2006, https://www.espn.com/espnmag/story?id=3644940.

24. Keating, "Doctor Yes."

25. Goldberg, "Concussions, Professional Sports, and Conflicts of Interest."

26. "Legal Issues Relating to Football Head Injuries (Part I & II): Hearings Before the Committee on the Judiciary House of Representatives, One Hundred Eleventh Congress, October 28, 2009 and January 4, 2010," Serial No. 111–82, p. 469, https://www.govinfo.gov/content/pkg/CHRG-111hhrg53092/html/CHRG-111hhrg53092.htm.

27. "Legal Issues Relating to Football Head Injuries," 30.

28. "Legal Issues Relating to Football Head Injuries," 85.

29. "Legal Issues Relating to Football Head Injuries," 85.

30. "Legal Issues Relating to Football Head Injuries," 86.

31. "Legal Issues Relating to Football Head Injuries," 86.

32. "Legal Issues Relating to Football Head Injuries," 87.

33. "Legal Issues Relating to Football Head Injuries," 110.

34. "Legal Issues Relating to Football Head Injuries," 110.

35. Kerianne H. Quanstrum and Rodney A. Hayward, "Lessons from the Mammography Wars," *New England Journal of Medicine* 363, no. 11 (2010): 1076–1079.

36. "Legal Issues Relating to Football Head Injuries," 116.

37. "Legal Issues Relating to Football Head Injuries," 116.

38. "Legal Issues Relating to Football Head Injuries," 116.

39. "Legal Issues Relating to Football Head Injuries," 118.

40. "Legal Issues Relating to Football Head Injuries," 2.

41. "Legal Issues Relating to Football Head Injuries," 334.

42. "Legal Issues Relating to Football Head Injuries," 363.

43. Faith Karimi and Emily Smith, "UNC Coach Under Fire Over His Remarks on Football's Link to Brain Illness," CNN.com, July 19, 2018, https://www.cnn.com/2018/07/19/health/larry-fedora-unc-cte-football/index.html.

44. Elizabeth Chuck, "Despite Evidence, Skeptics Try to Cast Doubt on CTE-Football Link," *NBC News*, August 30, 2018, https://www.nbcnews.com/news/sports/despite-evidence-skeptics-try-cast-doubt-cte-football-link-n897416.

45. Chuck, "Despite Evidence."

46. Steve Fainaru and Mark Fainaru-Wada, "Latest Studies: Brain Disease from Contact Sports More Common," *ESPN: Outside the Lines*, March 15, 2016, https://www.espn.com/espn/otl/story/_/id/14982032/nfl-admission-football-lead-brain

-disease-came-amid-new-science-suggesting-sports-related-trauma-becoming-more -common.

47. Fainaru and Fainaru-Wada, "Latest Studies."

48. See, e.g., Ann C. McKee, Jesse Mez, Bobak Abdolmohammadi, Morgane Butler, Bertrand Russell Huber, Madeline Uretsky, Katharine Babcock et al., "Neuro-pathologic and Clinical Findings in Young Contact Sport Athletes Exposed to Repetitive Head Impacts," *JAMA Neurology* (2023), August 28, 2023, doi:10.1001/jamaneurol .2023.2907; Kevin F. Bieniek, Melissa M. Blessing, Michael G. Heckman, Nancy N. Diehl, Amanda M. Serie, Michael A. Paolini II, Bradley F. Boeve et al., "Association Between Contact Sports Participation and Chronic Traumatic Encephalopathy: A Retrospective Cohort Study," *Brain Pathology* 30, no. 1 (2020): 63–74; Ann C. McKee, Michael L. Alosco, and Bertrand R. Huber, "Repetitive Head Impacts and Chronic Traumatic Encephalopathy," *Neurosurgery Clinics of North America* 27, no. 4 (2016): 529–535.

49. Thor D. Stein, Victor E. Alvarez, and Ann C. McKee, "Concussion in Chronic Traumatic Encephalopathy," *Current Pain and Headache Reports* 19 (2015): 1–6.

50. Daniel Engber and Stefan Fatsis, "Did *League of Denial* Get It Right?," *Slate*, October 11, 2013, https://slate.com/culture/2013/10/league-of-denial-dan-engber -and-stefan-fatsis-debate-the-frontline-documentary-on-the-nfl-and-concussions .html.

51. Zachary O. Binney and Kathleen E. Bachynski, "Estimating the Prevalence at Death of CTE Neuropathology among Professional Football Players," *Neurology* 92, no. 1 (2019): 43–45.

52. Jessica LeClair, Jennifer Weuve, Matthew P. Fox, Jesse Mez, Michael L. Alosco, Chris Nowinski, Ann McKee et al., "Relationship between Level of American Football Playing and Diagnosis of Chronic Traumatic Encephalopathy in a Selection Bias Analysis," *American Journal of Epidemiology* 191, no. 8 (2022): 1429–1443, quote at p. 1439.

53. LeClair et al., "Relationship between Level"; see also Christopher J. Nowinski, Samantha C. Bureau, Michael E. Buckland, Maurice A. Curtis, Daniel H. Daneshvar, Richard L. M. Faull, Lea T. Grinberg et al., "Applying the Bradford Hill Criteria for Causation to Repetitive Head Impacts and Chronic Traumatic Encephalopathy," *Frontiers in Neurology* 13 (2022): 938163 (citing studies).

54. See Sergio Sismondo, "Ghost Management: How Much of the Medical Literature Is Shaped Behind the Scenes by the Pharmaceutical Industry?," *PLOS Medicine* 4, no. 9 (2007): e286.

55. See, e.g., Erick H. Turner, "Publication Bias, with a Focus on Psychiatry: Causes and Solutions," *CNS Drugs* 27 (2013): 457–468; Joel Lexchin, Lisa A. Bero, Benjamin Djulbegovic, and Otavio Clark, "Pharmaceutical Industry Sponsorship

and Research Outcome and Quality: Systematic Review," *BMJ* 326, no. 7400 (2003): 1167–1170; Alison Thornton and Peter Lee, "Publication Bias in Meta-Analysis: Its Causes and Consequences," *Journal of Clinical Epidemiology* 53, no. 2 (2000): 207–216.

56. Bennet I. Omalu, Steven T. DeKosky, Ryan L. Minster, M. Ilyas Kamboh, Ronald L. Hamilton, and Cyril H. Wecht, "Chronic Traumatic Encephalopathy in a National Football League Player," *Neurosurgery* 57, no. 1 (2005): 128–134.

57. Ira R. Casson, Elliot J. Pellman, and David C. Viano, Comment on "Chronic Traumatic Encephalopathy in a National Football League Player," *Neurosurgery* 58, no. 5 (2006): E1152.

58. Casson, Pellman, and Viano, Comment on "Chronic Traumatic Encephalopathy."

59. Kenneth C. Kutner, Comment on "Chronic Traumatic Encephalopathy in a National Football League Player," *Neurosurgery* 58, no. 5 (2006): E1003.

60. Aaron Gordon, "The NFL, the NIH, and the Complications of Public-Private Scientific Research," *VICE*, December 7, 2016, https://www.vice.com/en/article/wnmgj4/nfl-nih-and-the-complications-of-public-private-scientific-research.

61. Gordon, "The NFL, the NIH."

62. Gordon, "The NFL, the NIH."

63. Steve Fainaru and Mark Fainaru-Wada, "NFL Health Officials Confronted NIH about Researcher Selection," *ESPN: Outside the Lines*, January 20, 2016, https://www.espn.com/espn/otl/story/_/id/14609331/nfl-says-did-not-intervene-nih-study-selection-nih-official-says-three-league-members-tried-do-so.

64. See Dominique A. Tobbell, *Pills, Power, and Policy: The Struggle for Drug Reform in Cold War America and Its Consequences* (Berkeley: University of California Press, 2012).

65. Bachynski and Goldberg, "Time Out," 180–181.

66. Bachynski and Goldberg, "Time Out," 181.

67. Bachynski and Goldberg, "Time Out," 181.

68. Bachynski and Goldberg, "Time Out," 181.

69. Mark Fainaru-Wada and Steve Fainaru, "NFL Retakes Control of Brain Research as Touted Alliance Ends," *ESPN: Outside the Lines*, August 31, 2017, https://www.espn.com/espn/otl/story/_/id/20509977/nfl-takes-control-brain-research-100-million-donation-all-ending-partnerships-entities.

70. Fainaru-Wada and Fainaru, "NFL Retakes Control."

71. Chad Arnold, "New York Lawmakers Are Considering a Ban on Tackle Football for Kids Under 12," *USA Today*, October 31, 2019, https://www.usatoday.com/story/news/nation/2019/10/31/new-york-considers-ban-youth-tackle-football-sparks-cte-debate/4107795002/.

72. Jerry L. Mashaw and David L. Harfst, *The Struggle for Auto Safety* (Cambridge, MA: Harvard University Press, 1990).

73. Bjørn Hofmann, "Is There a Technological Imperative in Health Care?," *International Journal of Technology Assessment in Health Care* 18, no. 3 (2002): 675–689; David J. Rothman, *Beginnings Count: The Technological Imperative in American Health Care* (New York: Oxford University Press, 1997).

74. Kathleen E. Bachynski, *No Game for Boys to Play: The History of Youth Football and the Origins of a Public Health Crisis* (Chapel Hill: University of North Carolina Press, 2019): 61.

75. Bachynski, *No Game for Boys to Play*, 61.

76. Kathleen E. Bachynski, "'The Duty of Their Elders'—Doctors, Coaches, and the Framing of Youth Football's Health Risks, 1950s–1960s," *Journal for the History of Medicine and Allied Sciences* 74, no. 2 (2019): 167–191.

77. Bachynski, "Duty of Their Elders."

78. Kathleen E. Bachynski and Daniel S. Goldberg, "Youth Sports & Public Health: Framing Risks of Mild Traumatic Brain Injury in American Football and Ice Hockey," *Journal of Law, Medicine & Ethics* 42, no. 3 (2014): 323–333, quote on pp. 325–326.

79. Bachynski, "Duty of Their Elders," 141.

80. Bachynski, "Duty of Their Elders," 141.

81. Bachynski, "Duty of Their Elders," 139.

82. Bachynski, "Duty of Their Elders," 140.

83. Bachynski, "Duty of Their Elders," 140.

84. Bachynski, "Duty of Their Elders," 145.

85. Alan Schwarz, "As Injuries Rise, Scant Oversight of Helmet Safety," *New York Times*, October 20, 2010, https://www.nytimes.com/2010/10/21/sports/football/21helmets.html.

86. Bachynski, *No Game for Boys to Play*, 24.

87. National Operating Committee on Standards for Athletic Equipment (NOCSAE), "FAQs: Does Certification to the NOCSAE Standard Mean That a Helmet Prevents Concussions?," https://nocsae.org/about-nocsae/faqs/#twentytwo (last accessed October 15, 2023).

88. Vicis, "FAQ: Is the Helmet Safer than Other Helmets? Will It Prevent Concussions?," https://web.archive.org/web/20200418165304/vicis.com/faq (last accessed October 6, 2023).

89. Historically, labor unions are immensely important players in both public health and, more specifically, in opposing regulated industries' efforts to manufacture doubt. The Manufacture of Doubt is a social octopus, stretching across vast swaths of social life, and hence it is not possible in a relatively short book to cover all

aspects of the script. Moreover, given this book's focus on vulnerable *nonemployee* participants in tackle football (i.e., youths and adolescents), the complex story of the tackle football labor union's role in worker health and brain injury must be reserved for additional work. For the history of labor unions in contesting agnotology and the Manufacture of Doubt, see in particular the work of David Rosner, Gerald Markowitz, Gerald Oppenheimer, James Colgrove, and Amy Fairchild. For the history of unions and public health in general, see the work of e.g., Ted Brown, Beatrix Hoffman, and Alondra Nelson.

90. Bachynski and Goldberg, "Youth Sports & Public Health, 323.

91. Bachynski and Goldberg, "Youth Sports & Public Health," 323–324.

Chapter 4. Conflicts of Interest and the Tackle Football Industry

1. Dominique A. Tobbell, *Pills, Power, and Policy: The Struggle for Drug Reform in Cold War America and Its Consequences* (Berkeley: University of California Press, 2012); Dominique A. Tobbell, "'Who's Winning the Human Race?' Cold War as Pharmaceutical Political Strategy," *Journal of the History of Medicine and Allied Sciences* 64, no. 4 (2009): 429–473; Dominique A. Tobbell, "Allied Against Reform: Pharmaceutical Industry–Academic Physician Relations in the United States, 1945–1970," *Bulletin of the History of Medicine* (2008): 878–912.

2. Tobbell, "Allied Against Reform," 881–882.

3. Tobbell, "Allied Against Reform," 882.

4. Tobbell, "Allied Against Reform," 884.

5. The sources are legion, but the canonical text is Paul Starr, *The Social Transformation of American Medicine: The Rise of a Sovereign Profession and the Making of a Vast Industry* (New York: Basic Books, 1982).

6. Tobbell, "Allied Against Reform," 898.

7. Tobbell, "Allied Against Reform," 900.

8. Tobbell, "Allied Against Reform," 900–901.

9. Tobbell, "Allied Against Reform," 902.

10. Tobbell, *Pills, Power, and Policy*, 9.

11. Tobbell, *Pills, Power, and Policy*, 9.

12. Andrew Stark, *Conflict of Interest in American Public Life* (Cambridge, MA: Harvard University Press, 2003). For discussion and extension of Stark's work to the health professions, see Daniel S. Goldberg "The Shadows of Sunlight: Why Disclosure Should Not Be a Priority in Addressing Conflicts of Interest," *Public Health Ethics* 12, no. 2 (2019): 202–212.

13. Alanna Durkin Richer, "Jury Says Drug Firm Founder Guilty of Bribing Doctors to Push Opioid," *PBS News Hour*, May 2, 2019, https://www.pbs.org/newshour /health/jury-says-drug-firm-founder-guilty-of-bribing-doctors-to-push-opioid.

14. Daniel S. Goldberg, "On Physician–Industry Relationships and Unreasonable Standards of Proof for Harm: A Population-Level Bioethics Approach," *Kennedy Institute of Ethics Journal* 26, no. 2 (2016): 173–194.

15. See, e.g., Lisa Cosgrove and Emily E. Wheeler, "Drug Firms, the Codification of Diagnostic Categories, and Bias in Clinical Guidelines," *Journal of Law, Medicine & Ethics* 41, no. 3 (2013): 644–653; Sunita Sah, "Conflicts of Interest and Your Physician: Psychological Processes That Cause Unexpected Changes in Behavior," *Journal of Law, Medicine & Ethics* 40, no. 3 (2012): 482–487; Christopher Robertson, Susannah Rose, and Aaron S. Kesselheim, "Effect of Financial Relationships on the Behaviors of Health Care Professionals: A Review of the Evidence," *Journal of Law, Medicine & Ethics* 40, no. 3 (2012): 452–466; Marc Rodwin, *Conflicts of Interest and the Future of Medicine: The United States, France, and Japan* (New York: Oxford University Press, 2011); Howard Brody, *Hooked: Ethics, the Medical Profession, and the Pharmaceutical Industry* (Lanham, MD: Rowman & Littlefield, 2007); Morten Andersen, Jakob Kragstrup, and Jens Søndergaard, "How Conducting a Clinical Trial Affects Physicians' Guideline Adherence and Drug Preferences," *JAMA* 295, no. 23 (2006): 2759–2764; Jason Dana and George Loewenstein, "A Social Science Perspective on Gifts to Physicians from Industry," *JAMA* 290, no. 2 (2003): 252–255; Mary-Margaret Chren and C. Seth Landefeld, "Physicians' Behavior and Their Interactions with Drug Companies: A Controlled Study of Physicians Who Requested Additions to a Hospital Drug Formulary," *JAMA* 271, no. 9 (1994): 684–689.

16. Jessica Bresler and Michael S. Sinha, "The Other Three Waves: Re-assessing the Impact of Industry–Prescriber Relations on the Opioid Crisis," *Journal of Legal Medicine* 41, no. 1–2 (2021): 47–81.

17. Goldberg, "On Physician-Industry Relationships and Unreasonable Standards of Proof."

18. David Michaels, *Doubt Is Their Product: How Industry's Assault on Science Threatens Your Health* (New York: Oxford University Press, 2008).

19. See sources cited in chapter 2, e.g, Sarah Milov, *The Cigarette: A Political History* (Cambridge, MA: Harvard University Press, 2019); Robert Proctor, *Golden Holocaust: Origins of the Cigarette Catastrophe and the Case for Abolition* (Berkeley: University of California Press, 2012); Allan Brandt, *The Cigarette Century: The Rise, Fall, and Deadly Persistence of the Product That Defined America* (New York: Basic Books, 2009).

20. Ilona Kickbusch, Luke Allen, and Christian Franz, "The Commercial Determinants of Health," *Lancet Global Health* 4, no. 12 (2016): e895–e896, quote on p. e895.

21. Melissa Mialon, "An Overview of the Commercial Determinants of Health," *Globalization and Health* 16 (2020): 1–7.

22. See Anna B. Gilmore, Alice Fabbri, Fran Baum, Adam Bertscher, Krista Bondy, Ha-Joon Chang, Sandro Demaio et al., "Defining and Conceptualising the Commercial Determinants of Health," *The Lancet* 401, no. 10383 (2023): 1194–1213; Mialon, "An Overview of the Commercial Determinants of Health."

23. Cecília Tomori, "Protecting, Promoting and Supporting Breastfeeding in All Policies: Reframing the Narrative," *Frontiers in Public Health* 11 (2023): 1149384.

24. Christopher R. Deubert, I. Glenn Cohen, and Holly Fernandez Lynch, "Protecting and Promoting the Health of NFL Players: Legal and Ethical Analysis and Recommendations," *The Football Players Health Study at Harvard University*, November 1, 2016, https://footballplayershealth.harvard.edu/wp-content/uploads/2016/11/01_Full_Report.pdf.

25. Mark Fainaru-Wada and Steve Fainaru, *League of Denial: The NFL, Concussions, and the Battle for Truth* (United States, Crown: 2014).

26. "Legal Issues Relating to Football Head Injuries (Part I & II): Hearings Before the Committee on the Judiciary House of Representatives, One Hundred Eleventh Congress, October 28, 2009 and January 4, 2010," Serial No. 111–82, p. 44, https://www.govinfo.gov/content/pkg/CHRG-111hhrg53092/html/CHRG-111hhrg53092.htm.

27. Judy Battista and Richard Sandomir, "League to Add Independent Trainer at Each Game to Check for Concussions," *New York Times*, December 20, 2011.

28. Daniel S. Goldberg, "Concussions, Professional Sports, and Conflicts of Interest: Why the National Football League's Current Policies Are Bad for Its (Players') Health," *HEC Forum* 20 (2008): 337–355, quote on pp. 343–344.

29. Deubert, Cohen, and Lynch, "Protecting and Promoting the Health of NFL Players," 99.

30. Deubert, Cohen, and Lynch, "Protecting and Promoting the Health of NFL Players," 99, Recommendation 2:1-A.

31. See Goldberg, "Shadows of Sunlight"; Arthur Schafer, "Biomedical Conflicts of Interest: A Defence of the Sequestration Thesis—Learning from the Cases of Nancy Olivieri and David Healy," *Journal of Medical Ethics* 30, no. 1 (2004): 8–24.

32. Deubert, Cohen, and Lynch, "Protecting and Promoting the Health of NFL Players," 124.

33. Howard Brody, "Professional Medical Organizations and Commercial Conflicts of Interest: Ethical Issues," *Annals of Family Medicine* 8, no. 4 (2010): 354–358, quote on p. 355.

34. Nathan Kalman-Lamb and Derek Silva, "'The Coaches Always Make the Health Decisions': Conflict of Interest as Exploitation in Power Five College Football," *SSM-Qualitative Research in Health* 5 (2024): 100405; Christine M. Baugh, Emily Kroshus, William P. Meehan, and Eric G. Campbell, "Trust, Conflicts of Interest, and

Concussion Reporting in College Football Players," *Journal of Law, Medicine & Ethics* 48, no. 2 (2020): 307–314.

35. Baugh et al., "Trust, Conflicts of Interest, and Concussion Reporting," 308.

36. This book is not principally focused on the COVID-19 pandemic. Although the pandemic unquestionably reveals much regarding attitudes towards youth and adolescent health in general, excavating the impact of COVID-19 and its relationship to collision sports and participation is easily another book in itself. Its relative omission from the analysis here is not a comment on the significance of the pandemic in general.

37. Bart Peterson, "Appropriate Medical Care Standards for High School Athletes," National Federation of State High School Associations, January 8, 2019, https://www.nfhs.org/articles/appropriate-medical-care-standards-for-high-school -athletes/.

38. Jeff G. Konin, Barbara J. Morris, Karen Liller, Andrew Carey, Eric Coris, and Michele Pescasio, "Status of Medical Coverage for High School Football Games in Florida," *Athletic Training & Sports Health Care* 3, no. 5 (2011): 226–229; Pietro M. Tonino and Matthew J. Bollier, "Medical Supervision of High School Football in Chicago: Does Inadequate Staffing Compromise Healthcare?," *Physician and Sportsmedicine* 32, no. 2 (2004): 37–40.

39. Terry L. DeWitt, Scott A. Unruh, and Srivatsa Seshadri, "The Level of Medical Services and Secondary School-Aged Athletes," *Journal of Athletic Training* 47, no. 1 (2012): 91–95.

Chapter 5. Unreasonable Demands for Proof of Causation and the Precautionary Principle

1. This chapter develops and extends the analysis of Daniel S. Goldberg, "What Does the Precautionary Principle Demand of Us: Ethics, Population Health Policy, and Sports-Related TBI," in *Sociocultural Examinations of Sports Concussions*, ed. Mary McDonald and Matt Ventresca (Taylor & Francis, 2019): 78–93.

2. Elihu D. Richter, Richard Laster, and Colin Soskolne, "The Precautionary Principle, Epidemiology and the Ethics of Delay," *Human and Ecological Risk Assessment: An International Journal* 11, no. 1 (2005): 17–27, quote on p. 18.

3. Daniel Steel, *Philosophy and the Precautionary Principle: Science, Evidence, and Environmental Policy* (Cambridge: Cambridge University Press, 2015).

4. Steel, *Philosophy and the Precautionary Principle*, 12.

5. Steel, *Philosophy and the Precautionary Principle*, 12.

6. "Introduction to Epidemiology," Centers for Disease Control, November 15, 2018, https://www.cdc.gov/training/publichealth101/epidemiology.html.

7. See, e.g., Jason Grossman and Fiona J. Mackenzie, "The Randomized Controlled Trial: Gold Standard, or Merely Standard?" *Perspectives in Biology and Medicine* 48, no. 4 (2005): 516–534.

8. Goldberg, "What Does the Precautionary Principle Demand of Us"; Daniel S. Goldberg, "On Physician–Industry Relationships and Unreasonable Standards of Proof for Harm: A Population-Level Bioethics Approach," *Kennedy Institute of Ethics Journal* 26, no. 2 (2016): 173–194.

9. Jan P. Vandenbroucke, Alex Broadbent, and Neil Pearce, "Causality and Causal Inference in Epidemiology: The Need For a Pluralistic Approach," *International Journal of Epidemiology* 45, no. 6 (2016): 1776–1786; see also Daniel S. Goldberg, "The Philosophical Implications of Fundamental Cause Theory," in *The Routledge Handbook of Philosophy of Public Health*, ed. Alex Broadbent and Sridhar Venkatapuram (Taylor & Francis, 2022).

10. Christopher J. Nowinski, Samantha C. Bureau, Michael E. Buckland, Maurice A. Curtis, Daniel H. Daneshvar, Richard L. M. Faull, Lea T. Grinberg et al., "Applying the Bradford Hill Criteria for Causation to Repetitive Head Impacts and Chronic Traumatic Encephalopathy," *Frontiers in Neurology* 13 (2022): 938163.

11. Nowinski et al., "Applying the Bradford Hill Criteria," 12.

12. Nowinski et al., "Applying the Bradford Hill Criteria," 3–5.

13. Nowinski et al., "Applying the Bradford Hill Criteria," 12.

14. Nowinski et al., "Applying the Bradford Hill Criteria," 12.

15. Goldberg, "What Does the Precautionary Principle Demand of Us"; Goldberg, "On Physician–Industry Relationships"; Douglas L. Weed, "Precaution, Prevention, and Public Health Ethics," *Journal of Medicine and Philosophy* 29, no. 3 (2004): 313–332.

16. See Alexandra Minna Stern, *Eugenic Nation: Faults and Frontiers of Better Breeding in Modern America* (Berkeley: University of California Press, 2016); Martin S. Pernick, "Eugenics and Public Health in American History," *American Journal of Public Health* 87, no. 11 (1997): 1767–1772.

17. Lawrence O. Gostin and Lindsay F. Wiley, *Public Health Law: Power, Duty, Restraint*, 3rd ed. (Berkeley: University of California Press, 2016).

18. "Legal Issues Relating to Football Head Injuries (Part I & II): Hearings Before the Committee on the Judiciary House of Representatives, One Hundred Eleventh Congress, October 28, 2009 and January 4, 2010," Serial No. 111–82, p. 116.

19. Jason Chung, Peter Cummings, and Uzma Samadani, "Questioning the Link Between Sports-Related Concussions and CTE," *The Health Care Blog*, February 12, 2018, https://thehealthcareblog.com/blog/2018/02/12/questioning-the-link-between-sports-related-concussions-and-cte/.

20. Jon S. Patricios, Kathryn J. Schneider, Jiri Dvorak, Osman Hassan Ahmed, Cheri Blauwet, Robert C. Cantu, Gavin A. Davis et al., "Consensus Statement on

Concussion in Sport: The 6th International Conference on Concussion in Sport–Amsterdam, October 2022," *British Journal of Sports Medicine* 57, no. 11 (2023): 695–711, quote on p. 705.

21. Patricios et al., "Consensus Statement on Concussion in Sport."

22. Uzma Samadani, Robert Glatter, Vikalpa Dammavalam, Vivian Papas, JeYeong Sone, and Abdullah Bin Zahid, *The Football Decision: An Exploration into Every Parent's Decision Whether or Not to Let a Child Play Contact Sports* (2015). Curiously, this book now seems almost completely unavailable for purchase; even Worldcat does not return holdings for the book. Samadani did give several public presentations surrounding the release of the book, including a keynote speech and participation in a podcast. See Uzma Samadani, "The Football Decision," keynote presentation at Minnesota Football Coaches Association annual meeting, 2016, Greg Spahn YouTube channel, https://www.youtube.com/watch?v=4L9P91ai7Jw.

23. This is an oversimplification, but to begin, see John Capps, "The Pragmatic Theory of Truth," *Stanford Encyclopedia of Philosophy*, Summer 2023 ed., ed. Edward N. Zalta and Uri Nodelman, https://plato.stanford.edu/archives/sum2023/entries/truth-pragmatic/; Richard Rorty, "Pragmatism, Davidson and Truth," in *Truth and Interpretation: Perspectives on the Philosophy of Donald Davidson*, ed. Ernest LePore (Blackwell: 1986): 333–355.

24. Zachary O. Binney and Kathleen E. Bachynski, "Estimating the Prevalence at Death of CTE Neuropathology among Professional Football Players," *Neurology* 92, no. 1 (2019): 43–45.

25. "Focus on Traumatic Brain Injury Research," NINDS, https://www.ninds.nih.gov/current-research/focus-disorders/focus-traumatic-brain-injury-research, accessed February 4, 2024.

26. CDC Heads Up, "Answering Questions About Chronic Traumatic Encephalopathy," CDC, January 2019, https://stacks.cdc.gov/view/cdc/78866.

27. Adam M. Finkel and Kevin F. Bieniek, "A Quantitative Risk Assessment for Chronic Traumatic Encephalopathy (CTE) in Football: How Public Health Science Evaluates Evidence," *Human and Ecological Risk Assessment: An International Journal* 25, no. 3 (2019): 564–589.

28. Finkel and Bieniek, "Quantitative Risk Assessment," 580.

29. Finkel and Bieniek, "Quantitative Risk Assessment," 580.

30. Goldberg, "On Physician–Industry Relationships," 185.

31. Goldberg, "What Does the Precautionary Principle Demand of Us," 88.

32. Yvonne M. Golightly, Stephen W. Marshall, Leigh F. Callahan, and Kevin Guskiewicz, "Early-Onset Arthritis in Retired National Football League Players," *Journal of Physical Activity and Health* 6, no. 5 (2009): 638–643.

33. Erik Poulsen, Glaucia H. Goncalves, Alessio Bricca, Ewa M. Roos, Jonas B.

Thorlund, and Carsten B. Juhl, "Knee Osteoarthritis Risk Is Increased 4–6 Fold after Knee Injury—A Systematic Review and Meta-analysis," *British Journal of Sports Medicine* 53, no. 23 (2019): 1454–1463.

34. Janet E. Simon and Carrie L. Docherty, "Current Health-Related Quality of Life in Former National Collegiate Athletic Association Division I Collision Athletes Compared with Contact and Limited-Contact Athletes," *Journal of Athletic Training* 51, no. 3 (2016): 205–212; Janet E. Simon and Carrie L. Docherty, "Current Health-Related Quality of Life Is Lower in Former Division I Collegiate Athletes than in Non–Collegiate Athletes," *American Journal of Sports Medicine* 42, no. 2 (2014): 423–429.

35. Simon and Docherty, "Current Health-Related Quality of Life," 208.

36. Linda B. Cottler, Arbi Ben Abdallah, Simone M. Cummings, John Barr, Rayna Banks, and Ronnie Forchheimer, "Injury, Pain, and Prescription Opioid Use among Former National Football League (NFL) Players," *Drug and Alcohol Dependence* 116, no. 1–3 (2011): 188–194.

37. Simon and Docherty, "Current Health-Related Quality of Life," 210.

Chapter 6. Policy Recommendations

1. Kathleen E. Bachynski and Daniel S. Goldberg, "Youth Sports & Public Health: Framing Risks of Mild Traumatic Brain Injury in American Football and Ice Hockey," *Journal of Law, Medicine & Ethics* 42, no. 3 (2014): 323–333.

2. Bachynski and Goldberg, "Youth Sports & Public Health," 331.

3. See, e.g., Jason A. Smith, "Law as a Social Determinant of Health," in *Public Health Law: Concepts and Case Studies*, ed. Montrece Ransom and Laura Magaña Valladeres (Springer, 2021): 257–266; Ruqaiijah Yearby, "Structural Racism and Health Disparities: Reconfiguring the Social Determinants of Health Framework to Include the Root Cause," *Journal of Law, Medicine & Ethics* 48, no. 3 (2020): 518–526; Wendy E. Parmet, "Immigration Law as a Social Determinant of Health," *Temple Law Review* 92 (2019): 931; Scott Burris, "From Health Care Law to the Social Determinants of Health: A Public Health Law Research Perspective," *University of Pennsylvania Law Review* 159, no. 6 (2011): 1649–1667; Scott Burris, "Law in a Social Determinants Strategy: A Public Health Law Research Perspective," *Public Health Reports* 126, no. 3_suppl (2011): 22–27.

4. Lawrence O. Gostin and Lindsay F. Wiley, *Public Health Law: Power, Duty, Restraint*, 3rd ed. (Berkeley: University of California Press, 2016), 4.

5. Gostin and Wiley, *Public Health Law*, 27.

6. Gostin and Wiley, *Public Health Law*, 27.

7. See, e.g., Alexander C. Wagenaar, Rosalie Liccardo Pacula, and Scott Burris, eds., *Legal Epidemiology: Theory and Methods*, 2nd ed. (Wiley, 2023); Scott Burris, Lindsay K. Cloud, and Matthew Penn, "The Growing Field of Legal Epidemiology,"

Journal of Public Health Management and Practice 26 (2020): S4–S9; Scott Burris, Marice Ashe, Donna Levin, Matthew Penn, and Michelle Larkin, "A Transdisciplinary Approach to Public Health Law: The Emerging Practice of Legal Epidemiology," *Annual Review of Public Health* 37 (2016): 135–148.

8. There are decades of research documenting the effects of structural racism on health outcomes; there is now emerging literature exploring the extent to which laws themselves are powerful mediators of these links. See, e.g., Madina Agénor, Carly Perkins, Catherine Stamoulis, Rahsaan D. Hall, Mihail Samnaliev, Stephanie Berland, and S. Bryn Austin, "Developing a Database of Structural Racism–Related State Laws for Health Equity Research and Practice in the United States," *Public Health Reports* 136, no. 4 (2021): 428–440.

9. Jingzhen Yang, Hosea H. Harvey, Lindsay Sullivan, Lihong Huang, and R. Dawn Comstock, "Association between Design Elements of Concussion Laws and Reporting of Sports-Related Concussions among US High School Athletes, 2009–2017," *Public Health Reports* 136, no. 6 (2021): 745–753; Lindsay Sullivan, Hosea H. Harvey, Gary A. Smith, and Jingzhen Yang, "Putting Policy into Practice: School-Level Compliance with and Implementation of State Concussion Laws," *Journal of Public Health Management and Practice* 26 (2020): S84–S92.

10. Christine Atherstone, Molly Siegel, Emily Schmitt-Matzen, Scott Sjoblom, Joy Jackson, Carina Blackmore, and John Neatherlin, "SARS-CoV-2 Transmission Associated with High School Wrestling Tournaments—Florida, December 2020– January 2021," *Morbidity and Mortality Weekly Report* 70, no. 4 (2021): 141.

11. Yang et al., "Association between Design Elements."

12. Madison Powers and Ruth Faden, *Social Justice: The Moral Foundations of Public Health and Health Policy* (New York: Oxford University Press, 2008).

13. Powers and Faden, *Social Justice*, 71.

14. Powers and Faden, *Social Justice*, 71; see also Daniel S. Goldberg, *Public Health Ethics and the Social Determinants of Health* (Springer, 2017), 17–32; Zackary D. Berger and Daniel S. Goldberg, "Caught in the Web—US Immigration and Compound Disadvantage," *New England Journal of Medicine* 381, no. 11 (2019): 993–995.

15. See Goldberg, *Public Health Ethics and the Social Determinants of Health*, 17–32.

16. Bruna Galobardes, Mary Shaw, Debbie A. Lawlor, John W. Lynch, and George Davey Smith, "Indicators of Socioeconomic Position (Part 1)," *Journal of Epidemiology and Community Health* 60, no. 1 (2006): 7–12.

17. Madison Powers and Ruth Faden, "Social Practices, Public Health and the Twin Aims of Justice: Responses to Comments," *Public Health Ethics* 6, no. 1 (2013): 45–49.

18. Chris Nowinski and Robert Cantu, "Flag Football under 14: An Education

Campaign for Parents," *Concussion Legacy Foundation*, February 2021, https://concussionfoundation.org/sites/default/files/2021-02/Flag_Under_14_White_Paper_110119.pdf.

19. Nowinski and Cantu, "Flag Football under 14," 4.

20. Nowinski and Cantu, "Flag Football under 14," 5.

21. Tyler J. Young, Ray W. Daniel, Steven Rowson, and Stefan M. Duma, "Head Impact Exposure in Youth Football: Elementary School Ages 7–8 Years and the Effect of Returning Players," *Clinical Journal of Sport Medicine* 24, no. 5 (2014): 416–421; Bryan R. Cobb, Jillian E. Urban, Elizabeth M. Davenport, Steven Rowson, Stefan M. Duma, Joseph A. Maldjian, Christopher T. Whitlow et al., "Head Impact Exposure in Youth Football: Elementary School Ages 9–12 Years and the Effect of Practice Structure," *Annals of Biomedical Engineering* 41 (2013): 2463–2473.

22. Nowinski and Cantu, "Flag Football under 14," 3.

23. Carolyn A. Emery, Paul Eliason, Vineetha Warriyar, Luz Palacios-Derflingher, Amanda Marie Black, Maciek Krolikowski, Nicole Spencer et al., "Body Checking in Non-Elite Adolescent Ice Hockey Leagues: It Is Never Too Late for Policy Change Aiming to Protect the Health of Adolescents," *British Journal of Sports Medicine* 56, no. 1 (2022): 12–17.

24. Daniel S. Goldberg, "Mild Traumatic Brain Injury, the National Football League, and the Manufacture of Doubt: An Ethical, Legal, and Historical Analysis," *Journal of Legal Medicine* 34, no. 2 (2013): 157–191, quote on pp. 170–171.

25. Goldberg, "Mild Traumatic Brain Injury, 170–171.

26. Colin M. MacLeod, "Conceptions of Parental Autonomy," *Politics & Society* 25, no. 1 (1997): 117–140; Steven Mintz, "Regulating the American Family," *Journal of Family History* 14, no. 4 (1989): 387–408.

27. Mintz, "Regulating the American Family," 388.

28. Mintz, "Regulating the American Family," 401.

29. Mintz, "Regulating the American Family," 402.

30. In addition, from a disability ethics perspective, there are countless moral problems with the idea that a child's particular body form is "defective" and requires repeated invasive interventions to correct. Critiquing this norm, and the medical model from which it flows, is rightly considered a point of departure in disability bioethics and perhaps in disability studies in general. See, e.g., Alicia Ouellette, *Bioethics and Disability: Towards a Disability-Conscious Bioethics* (Cambridge: Cambridge University Press, 2011); Jackie Leach Scully, *Disability Bioethics: Moral Bodies, Moral Difference* (Lanham, MD: Rowman & Littlefield, 2008).

31. United States v. Carroll Towing, 159 F.2d 169 (2nd Cir. 1947).

32. See Daniel Wikler and Dan W. Brock, "Population-Level Bioethics: Mapping a

New Agenda," in *Ethics, Prevention, and Public Health*, ed. Angus Dawson and Marcel Verweij (New York: Oxford University Press, 2007): 78–94.

33. William J. Winslade, *Confronting Traumatic Brain Injury: Devastation, Hope, and Healing* (New Haven, CT: Yale University Press, 1999).

34. Altaf Saadi, Sarah Bannon, Eric Watson, and Ana-Maria Vranceanu, "Racial and Ethnic Disparities associated with Traumatic Brain Injury across the Continuum of Care: A Narrative Review and Directions for Future Research," *Journal of Racial and Ethnic Health Disparities* 9 (2022): 786–799; Einat K. Brenner, Emily C. Grossner, Benjamin N. Johnson, Rachel A. Bernier, José Soto, and Frank G. Hillary, "Race and Ethnicity Considerations in Traumatic Brain Injury Research: Incidence, Reporting, and Outcome," *Brain Injury* 34, no. 6 (2020): 801–810.

35. Saadi et al., "Racial and Ethnic Disparities."

36. Brenner et al., "Race and Ethnicity Considerations in Traumatic Brain Injury," 801.

37. Staja Q. Booker, Emily J. Bartley, Keesha Powell-Roach, Shreela Palit, Calia Morais, Osheeca J. Thompson, Yenisel Cruz-Almeida et al., "The Imperative for Racial Equality in Pain Science: A Way Forward," *Journal of Pain* 22, no. 12 (2021): 1578–1585; Daniel S. Goldberg, *The Bioethics of Pain Management: Beyond Opioids* (Taylor & Francis, 2014), citing sources.

38. For a longer analysis of the implications of participation in American tackle football from a racial injustice perspective, see Goldberg, "Mild Traumatic Brain Injury," 183–189.

39. California Health and Safety Code § 124241 (2023).

40. "Healthcare Access in Rural Communities," Rural Health Information Hub, January 31, 2024, https://www.ruralhealthinfo.org/topics/healthcare-access.

41. "Healthcare Access in Rural Communities."

42. Martin MacDowell, Michael Glasser, Michael Fitts, Kimberly Nielsen, and Matthew Hunsaker, "A National View of Rural Health Workforce Issues in the USA," *Rural Remote Health* 10, no. 3 (2010): 1531.

43. This kind of flexibility is a basic feature of tort law and policy in the US. The tort law system often imposes objective standards, the subjective requirements for which vary with time, place, and circumstance. Thus, the basic standard for negligence requires actors to behave as a reasonably prudent person would behave under the same or similar set of circumstances. What constitutes reasonable behavior will vary depending on the exact circumstances, just as what constitutes a minimally sufficient level of health care services may vary.

44. Cecília Tomori, "Protecting, Promoting and Supporting Breastfeeding in All Policies: Reframing the Narrative," *Frontiers in Public Health* 11 (2023): 1149384;

Melissa Mialon, "An Overview of the Commercial Determinants of Health," *Globaiza-tion and Health* 16 (2020): 1–7; Ilona Kickbusch, Luke Allen, and Christian Franz, "The Commercial Determinants of Health," *Lancet Global Health* 4, no. 12 (2016): e895–e896.

45. Daniel S. Goldberg "The Shadows of Sunlight: Why Disclosure Should Not Be a Priority in Addressing Conflicts of Interest," *Public Health Ethics* 12, no. 2 (2019): 202–212; Daylian M. Cain, George Loewenstein, and Don A. Moore, "When Sunlight Fails to Disinfect: Understanding the Perverse Effects of Disclosing Conflicts of Interest," *Journal of Consumer Research* 37, no. 5 (2011): 836–857.

46. See Howard Brody, *Hooked: Ethics, the Medical Profession, and the Pharma-ceutical Industry* (Lanham, MD: Rowman & Littlefield, 2007): 321–326.

47. See Goldberg, "Shadows of Sunlight"; Arthur Schafer, "Biomedical Conflicts of Interest: A Defence of the Sequestration Thesis—Learning from the Cases of Nancy Olivieri and David Healy," *Journal of Medical Ethics* 30, no. 1 (2004): 8–24.

48. Cecília Tomori, "Scientists: Don't Feed the Doubt Machine," *Nature* 599, no. 7883 (2021): 9.

49. "WHO Statement on Philip Morris funded Foundation for a Smoke-Free World," September 28, 2017, World Health Organization website, https://www.who .int/news/item/28-09-2017-who-statement-on-philip-morris-funded-foundation-for -a-smoke-free-world.

50. "WHO Statement," citing WHO Framework Convention on Tobacco Control, "Guidelines for Implementation of Article 5.3," January 1, 2013, https://fctc.who.int /publications/m/item/guidelines-for-implementation-of-article-5.3.

51. Alan Finder, "At One University, Tobacco Money Is a Secret," *New York Times*, May 22, 2008, https://www.nytimes.com/2008/05/22/us/22tobacco.html.

52. Finder, "At One University."

53. Patrick Hruby, "Friday Night Lights Out: The Case for Abolishing High School Football," *VICE Sports*, November 29, 2016, https://www.vice.com/en/article /53xy8k/friday-night-lights-out-the-case-for-abolishing-high-school-football.

54. Randall Curren and J. C. Blokhuis, "Friday Night Lights Out: The End of Football in Schools," *Harvard Educational Review* 88, no. 2 (2018): 141–162, quote on pp. 142–143.

55. Scott M. Reid, "Mater Dei to Commission Independent Probe of Its Sports Programs," *Orange County Register*, November 30, 2021, https://www.ocregister.com /2021/11/30/mater-dei-to-commission-independent-probe-of-its-sports-programs/.

56. Reid, "Mater Dei to Commission Independent Probe."

57. Reid, "Mater Dei to Commission Independent Probe."

58. Reid, "Mater Dei to Commission Independent Probe."

59. Reid, "Mater Dei to Commission Independent Probe."

60. Scott M. Reid, Steve Fryer, and Dan Albano, "Mater Dei, Diocese of Orange

Won't Release Report on School's Athletic Culture," *Orange County Register*, January 18, 2023, https://www.ocregister.com/2023/01/18/mater-dei-diocese-of-orange-wont-release-report-on-schools-athletic-culture/.

61. Reid, "Mater Dei."

62. Reid, "Mater Dei to Commission Independent Probe."

63. Curren and Blokhuis, "Friday Night Lights Out," 146. These vices are also found even in games that aren't considered deep play if the sport draws political and social significance from other sources, such as international gymnastics. There is much to be said about the vices that flourished in the culture of US Gymnastics, some of which involved COIs and motivated bias among team physicians who also treated college football players.

64. Hruby, "Friday Night Lights Out."

65. Curren and Blokhuis, "Friday Night Lights Out," 145.

66. Curren and Blokhuis, "Friday Night Lights Out," 146, 147.

67. Curren and Blokhuis, "Friday Night Lights Out," 151.

68. Curren and Blokhuis, "Friday Night Lights Out," 150; see also J. C. Blokhuis, "Whose Custody Is It Anyway? 'Homeschooling' from a *Parens Patriae* Perspective," *Theory and Research in Education* 8, no. 2 (2010): 199–222.

69. See, e.g., Seth J. Prins, Sandhya Kajeepeta, Mark L. Hatzenbuehler, Charles C. Branas, Lisa R. Metsch, and Stephen T. Russell, "School Health Predictors of the School-to-Prison Pipeline: Substance Use and Developmental Risk and Resilience Factors," *Journal of Adolescent Health* 70, no. 3 (2022): 463–469.

70. Curren and Blokhuis, "Friday Night Lights Out," 154.

71. Christian M. Wade, "Bill to Ban Tackling in Youth Football Meets Backlash," *Eagle Tribune*, February 26, 2019, https://www.eagletribune.com/news/bill-to-ban-tackling-in-youth-football-meets-backlash/article_d6031695-a4d8-5e88-b81d-871c10c711f8.html.

72. Thomas Prohaska, "Morinello, Ortt, Coaches, Deride Bill That Would Ban Tackle Football Under Age 12," *Buffalo News*, November 9, 2019, https://buffalonews.com/news/local/morinello-ortt-coaches-deride-bill-that-would-ban-tackle-football-under-age-12/article_23173f67-2fe2-5c46-a5af-6fb9aab80538.html.

73. Jamila Michener, "A Racial Equity Framework for Assessing Health Policy," Commonwealth Fund, January 20, 2022, https://doi.org/10.26099/ejob-6g71.

74. Michener, "Racial Equity Framework."

75. Michener, "Racial Equity Framework."

76. For extensive discussion of this point, see Joan Benach, Davide Malmusi, Yutaka Yasui, José Miguel Martínez, and Carles Muntaner, "Beyond Rose's Strategies: A Typology of Scenarios of Policy Impact on Population Health and Health Inequalities," *International Journal of Health Services* 41, no. 1 (2011): 1–9.

77. Georgia F. Symons, Meaghan Clough, Joanne Fielding, William T. O'Brien, Claire E. Shepherd, David K. Wright, and Sandy R. Shultz, "The Neurological Consequences of Engaging in Australian Collision Sports," *Journal of Neurotrauma* 37, no. 5 (2020): 792–809, emphasis added.

78. William P. Meehan III, Alex M. Taylor, Paul Berkner, Noah J. Sandstrom, Mark W. Peluso, Matthew M. Kurtz, Alvaro Pascual-Leone et al., "Division III Collision Sports Are Not Associated with Neurobehavioral Quality of Life," *Journal of Neurotrauma* 33, no. 2 (2016): 254–259, quote on p. 255.

79. This is not to suggest that an outright ban is per se unethical. This argument is best made elsewhere; the point here is merely to show the relative weakness of the case for the proposed ban subsequent to successful implementation of Policy Recommendation #1.

80. Shira Springer, "WBUR Poll: For Head Injuries, Football Fans Support Regulation," WBUR, January 29, 2018, https://www.wbur.org/news/2018/01/29/wbur-poll-football-concussions.

81. Aletha Y. Akers, Melvin R. Muhammad, and Giselle Corbie-Smith, "'When You Got Nothing to Do, You Do Somebody': A Community's Perceptions of Neighborhood Effects on Adolescent Sexual Behaviors," *Social Science & Medicine* 72, no. 1 (2011): 91–99; Crystal W. Cené, Aletha Y. Akers, Stacey W. Lloyd, Tashuna Albritton, Wizdom Powell Hammond, and Giselle Corbie-Smith, "Understanding Social Capital and HIV Risk in Rural African American Communities," *Journal of General Internal Medicine* 26 (2011): 737–744; Nancy L. Fleischer, Ana V. Diez Roux, Marcio Alazraqui, and Hugo Spinelli, "Social Patterning of Chronic Disease Risk Factors in a Latin American City," *Journal of Urban Health* 85 (2008): 923–937; Graham Scambler and Sasha Scambler, "Social Patterning of Health Behaviours," in *Public Health: Social Context and Action*, ed. Angela Scriven and Sebastian Garman (McGraw Hill, 2007): 34–47; Martin J. Jarvis and Jane Wardle, "Social Patterning of Individual Health Behaviours: The Case of Cigarette Smoking," in *Social Determinants of Health*, 2nd ed., ed. Michael Marmot and Richard Wilkinson (New York: Oxford University Press, 2006): 224–237.

82. See Akers, Muhammad, and Corbie-Smith, "When You Got Nothing to Do"; Cené et al., "Understanding Social Capital and HIV Risk."

83. See Daniel S. Goldberg, "The Implications of Fundamental Cause Theory for Priority Setting," *American Journal of Public Health* 104, no. 10 (2014): 1839–1843.

84. Jayson L. Lusk and Anne Rozan, "Public Policy and Endogenous Beliefs: The Case of Genetically Modified Food," *Journal of Agricultural and Resource Economics* 33, no. 2 (2008): 270–289.

85. Kingdon's policy streams model is the subject of a considerable secondary

literature, but for the fundamentals, see John Kingdon, *Agendas, Alternatives, and Public Policy*, 2nd ed. (New York: Pearson, 2010).

Conclusion

1. Ayah Nuriddin, Graham Mooney, and Alexandre I. R. White, "Reckoning with Histories of Medical Racism and Violence in the USA," *The Lancet* 396, no. 10256 (2020): 949–951; Paul E. Farmer, Bruce Nizeye, Sara Stulac, and Salmaan Keshavjee, "Structural Violence and Clinical Medicine," *PLOS Medicine* 3, no. 10 (2006): e449; Paul Farmer, *Pathologies of Power: Health, Human Rights, and the New War on the Poor* (Berkeley: University of California Press, 2004). For an important recent contribution connecting concepts of structural violence to histories of injury, capitalism, and occupational harm, see Nate Holdren, *Injury Impoverished: Workplace Accidents, Capitalism, and Law in the Progressive Era* (Cambridge: Cambridge University Press, 2020).

2. Stephen T. Casper and Kelly O'Donnell, "The Punch-Drunk Boxer and the Battered Wife: Gender and Brain Injury Research," *Social Science & Medicine* 245 (2020): 112688.

3. T. Elon Dancy, Kirsten T. Edwards, and James Earl Davis, "Historically White Universities and Plantation Politics: Anti-Blackness and Higher Education in the Black Lives Matter Era," *Urban Education* 53, no. 2 (2018): 176–195; Billy Hawkins, *The New Plantation: Black Athletes, College Sports, and Predominantly White NCAA Institutions* (Springer, 2010).

4. Christina Gough, "Share of Head Coaches for Men's NCAA Division I Football Teams in the United States in 2022, By Ethnicity," Statista, March 29, 2023, https://www.statista.com/statistics/1375227/ncaa-division-i-football-head-coaches-ethnicity/.

5. Lindsay F. Wiley and Lawrence O. Gostin, *Public Health Law and Ethics: Power, Duty, Restraint*, 4th ed. (Berkeley: University of California Press, 2024), forthcoming.

Index

administrative law, 46–47
adolescents. *See* children and adolescents; high school and youth football
adverse childhood experiences, 27–28
agnotology, 51, 53–54, 74, 87, 106. *See also* Manufacture of Doubt
Air Hygiene Foundation, 47–48
antecedent acts, 112–13, 116, 120, 121, 176
arthritis. *See* inflammatory disease
asbestos, 16, 49, 66. *See also* silicosis
ASTM, 98
auto industry and driving, 6–7, 40, 94, 137

Bachynski, Kathleen E., 85–86, 91–92, 96–97, 98, 99, 100, 102, 141
Bailes, Julian, 82–83
Bailey, Pearce, 38
bans on tackling, 5–6, 93–94, 158–65, 184–86, 192, 194, 197
bans on youth football, 190–92, 195
Baugh, Christine M., 123
behavior of partiality, 112–13, 116, 120, 121–22, 176, 178–79
Bentham, Jeremy, 11
bias: defined, 105; publication, 87; selection, 85–86; towards the null, 142. *See also* conflicts of interest; motivated bias
Bieniek, Kevin F., 141–42, 143
Binney, Zachary O., 85–86, 141
Blokhuis, J. C., 177–78, 180–82, 183
Bornstein, Steve, 75
boxing, viii, 81, 82, 164, 177
Bradford Hill criteria, 133–34
brain: development, vii, 17, 158–59; and identity, 22. *See also* chronic traumatic encephalopathy; traumatic brain injuries
Bramwell, Wyatt, ix
Brenner, Einat K., 164–65
Brown & Williamson, 52, 60
Butler, Jon, 65–66

cancer, 27, 52–53, 57, 59–61, 77, 174
capitalism, racial, 13
Casson, Ira, 81, 88, 138
causal inference: plethora of evidence on TBIs, 41, 83–86, 141–48, 162–63, 181; tools for, 132–35, 143
causation, demands for proof of: by auto industry, 40; causal inference tools, 133–35, 143; central role of in Manufacture of Doubt, 9, 70, 137–38, 140, 196; and conflicts of interest, 104; by football industry, viii–ix, 9, 70, 74–83, 85, 138–39, 140, 144–46; general causation vs. causation in individuals, 61–62; plethora of evidence on TBIs, 41, 83–86, 141–48, 162–63, 181; by railroad industry, 40, 51, 59, 70; and randomized controlled trials, 130–32, 144, 145–46; and "reasonableness," 77–79, 132; and regulatory vacuum, 79, 142, 146, 148; and silicosis, 43–45, 51, 59, 70; study challenges, 21, 129–36; by tobacco industry, 52, 53–54, 58–62, 70, 77, 80. *See also* evidence focus
CDC Foundation, 91–92
Centers for Disease Control and Prevention (CDC), 91–92, 141
children and adolescents: adverse childhood experiences, 27–28; and brain development, vii, 17, 158–59; brain injuries, increase in, vii, ix; brain injuries, vulnerability to, 17, 26–29, 158–60; and informed consent, vii–viii, x, 28–29; and scope of population, 26–29. *See also* high school and youth football
chronic traumatic encephalopathy (CTE): Bradford Hill criteria, 134; and brain changes, 84–86; and causation language, 141; in Congressional hearings, 78, 81–82; defined, viii, 7–8; and denial of causation, 75, 78, 81–83, 85, 88, 138; diagnosis of, viii;